Erectile Dysfunction

*The Most Effective, Permanent
Solution to Finally Overcoming
Impotence and Sexual Dysfunction
for Your Sexual Health*

Bradley Martin

been made to provide accurate, up to date and reliable complete information. No warranties of any kind are expressed or implied. Readers acknowledge that the author is not engaging in the rendering of legal, financial, medical or professional advice.

By reading this document, the reader agrees that under no circumstances are we responsible for any losses, direct or indirect, which are incurred as a result of the use of information contained within this document, including, but not limited to, — errors, omissions, or inaccuracies.

Table of Contents

Introduction

If you are buying this book, then it may just be a lifesaver in the bedroom. Many people are unsure of what causes erectile dysfunction. This book explores all the avenues and leaves you with a clear idea of how to fix erectile dysfunction forever. The complex nature of something like this is that men find themselves in a very vulnerable situation. It's natural that a man will want to make love, and the body telling him that he cannot, can be one of the most difficult things that a man can go through.

This book delves into the ways you can follow up by learning more about why your penis will not remain sufficiently hard to perform. It may actually reveal secrets to you that you hadn't thought about. The act of sex depends on several things and the book goes into detail on each aspect of lovemaking that may affect the way that the penis reacts.

Once you understand more than just the mechanics of it, you will be able to see that no one's to blame and that the dysfunction that you are experiencing can be reversed. However, the solutions are not always obvious to a man. This is where a guide such as this helps. It explains options. It explains reasons and, most of all, does so in a no nonsense manner that's easy to understand.

Once you can get beyond your worries and learn why it's happening, you are half way to solving the problem forever. That's got to be worth it for you and for your partner. It isn't a question of being a failure as a man. It's a question of learning what you can do to make a permanent difference.

If you are a man with this problem, there are also many advantages to this book because it will teach you how the female of the species can also be of help to you and you will learn why she would want to. You need never be alone again with this dilemma. Having bought the book, you are already on the road to recovery and can get there easily by following the instructions in the book to a tee.

Your erectile dysfunction can be something of the past, and you can go on making love for years to come. It isn't the end of the road by a long chalk, but you will need to take account of all of the chapters, rather than just those that please you.

Important note: Although throughout this book, partners are referred to as 'she,' the advice is also applicable to male partners in most instances, unless a purely female perspective is more relevant. However, to ensure a good flow of writing and avoid any syntax disruption from repeatedly referring to 'he or she,' the author has chosen to use 'she' for the sake of flow and uniformity.

Chapter 1

How Erectile Dysfunction Can Affect Your Life

Erectile dysfunction is no silly or laughing matter. People may say a soft wiener isn't a life-altering problem like world peace, famine or nuclear warheads in the hands of terrorists but hey, it is for men who suffer from them and their partners. Believe it or not, erectile dysfunction can affect one's relationships.

A sexual relationship between a man and a woman is the most private relationship that anyone can ever get into and a man's inability to have or sustain erections can significantly alter his relationship with himself and his partner. For one, the man suffering from erectile dysfunction can suffer from feelings of guilt and embarrassment that can discourage him from opening up to the other person. Over time, the man may stop being vulnerable in other areas of his life as well and may lead to a widening rift between him and his woman.

Sex is critical in terms of keeping a marriage strong and healthy. Because erectile dysfunctions normally keep married couples from enjoying each other in the bedroom, it can affect greatly affect marriages over the long term. Some experts estimate that 20 percent of failed marriages can be traced to erectile dysfunctions. And failed marriages are no silly or laughing matter.

For couples that are affected by a man's erectile dysfunction, it starts with failed sexual advances. Over time, this can erode the couple's closeness, intimacy and trust. The man who suffers from erectile dysfunction may start to distance himself from the woman both physically and emotionally due to fear of being embarrassed by a limp wiener. In return, the woman may feel she is no longer desirable and that the man's passion for her is waning or ha already waned, which makes her feel unattractive and inferior.

In most cases, that's not the case. Men will usually want to have sex with their female partners but erectile dysfunction prevents them from doing so both by preventing full course sex (with penetration) or discouraging them from making advances at all. As stated earlier, it can affect the woman's own sense of self-esteem and intimacy with her man and as the cycle perpetuates itself, the relationship eventually deteriorates to the point that both partners' hearts have drifted away from each other.

Game over.

The women partners that are most vulnerable to being affected emotionally and psychologically by their male partner's erectile dysfunctions are those whose sense of self worth and attractiveness are hinged on how much their partners want to have sex with them. Because a hard wiener is just about the only objective way of validating how sexually desirable the man finds a woman, a soft wiener despite erotic advances by the woman will lead her to believe she's undesirable and unattractive to her man. From such feelings can come suspicions of infidelity as well.

Game over.

As erectile dysfunction continues to erode a couple's sexual intimacy, either or both partners may subconsciously seek revenge by withholding sex even more, further worsening the situation. The partners may start to seek fulfillment and joy from other things instead of each other.

Game over.

Erectile dysfunction doesn't just affect a man's romantic relationship – it can also affect the way he relates to other people, such as co-workers and friends. How so? Even if his penile issue doesn't directly get in the way of his non-romantic relationships, it can affect his self-esteem, morale and the ability to enjoy life. He may try to compensate externally by trying to look macho and virile but deep inside, he may be wasting away knowing he's impotent.

The same erosion in self-esteem and morale may lead to reduced work productivity. As those two continue to erode, it can also affect his view of himself as an employee, manager or entrepreneur, which can discourage him from giving it his best. And because erectile dysfunction is – for many people – a silly and laughing matter, a man may choose to keep it to himself and feel isolated from everyone.

To summarize, men are affected both psychologically and physically by erectile dysfunction. As the average male lifespan continues to increase, erectile dysfunction will become an even more important issue in their lives. As such, everyone should be sensitive to and realize that sexuality really is an important part of our lives.

Medical professionals must be able to develop skills to guide patients. Erectile dysfunction may involve more than one factor and as such, the ability to use different methods to address erectile dysfunction can go a long way towards resolving cases of such. Such multi-faceted approaches should consider the nuances of existing partnerships and relationships in order to effectively address erectile dysfunction.

Chapter 2

How Erectile Dysfunction Affects Your Partner

For many women partners of men who suffer from erectile dysfunction, the problem is a sexual one. This despite the fact that most causes of erectile dysfunction are anything but sexual. Ignorance of erectile dysfunction's true causes often worsen such women's feelings of low self-worth, unattractiveness, anxiety, hurt and even anger.

As mentioned earlier, erectile dysfunction, especially if the man isn't vulnerable enough with his female partner about it, can make the women feel either undesirable, that the man is having an affair or both. As this happens, women may start to confront the man about his inability to "stand up" by asking questions with some tone of anxiety, hurt or even anger.

Often times, the man suffering from erectile dysfunction may interpret such manner of asking as an affront or attack on his character and manhood and thus, worsens the situation by pulling further away emotionally and physically. His female partner may retaliate by pulling further away too, thinking that the man's response was a confirmation of her suspicions. As this happens, the female partner may feel even worse about herself and may open the door for anxiety or even depression to come barging into her heart and mind, bringing along with them an even stronger paranoid feeling. And the crazy cycle continues to spin out of control until...

Game over.

The Other Extreme

While many women react to their male partner's erectile dysfunction by pulling away, some go the other extreme: they go overboard in trying to seduce their male partners into "hardening up". With the belief that erectile dysfunction is merely a sexual issue, they think that sexing it up even more by trying to dress in the sexiest and kinkiest undies is the key to making their men "stand up" and take notice.

This approach, however, may be counterproductive. Why? Considering that erectile dysfunction isn't purely a sexual issue, the man may feel pressured to have his wiener as hard as a rock. As he feels even more anxious about his inability to "stand up", the more like his penis will remain flaccid.

The same thing will probably happen if the female partner tries to sex it up by becoming even more physical, say, stroking or sucking him harder. Because it's not necessarily about sex or the female partner, doing so will just make the man more anxious and stressed, keep his wiener soft and lead to greater frustration for the woman.

Can you see why erectile dysfunction is a serious matter indeed?

Chapter 3

Things That Affect Your Performance

The body is made up of different parts which each have their function. The penis is used for sexual contact and to reproduce. It's also made for being a vessel for urine. The penis area of a man is a very sensitive area, but erection happens because of various things:

Stimulation of the penis

The British Journal of Urology received a report as far back as 2009 that studies on healthy men found that stimulation points, which were common indicators of erection, were quite specific. Men were asked what trigger points helped them to get an erection. Most replies were consistent and the glans (or the end) of the penis was one of the most sensitive areas for most men. Just below the glans a super sensitive area exists where the foreskin is usually attached to the glans in men who have not been circumcised, but it was also found that this area was also super sensitive in the case of those who had been circumcised. It was quite a surprise that areas that researchers thought may have been good stimulation points were not that high on the list.

The scrotum area, the nipples and the neck were not areas that made a man particularly erect. Thus it can be seen that the penis itself needs the stimulation or that thoughts directly related to the penis by the man stimulated by external triggers will direct themselves on the flow of blood to the penis.

In the case of erectile dysfunction this doesn't happen so well.

What an erection is

An erection is when a signal is sent to the penis from the brain to tell it that penile blood vessels need to relax. It is this relaxation of the blood vessels that allow the flow of blood into the penis. This is then trapped within the penis to sustain erection.

From the above definition, you can see that an erection consists of several actions:

- Thought

- Message from brain to penis

- Blood flow

- Trapping the excess blood in the penis

It sounds pretty basic and simple, but it's not. For the mind to send the message to the penis, it has to feel stimulated. For the blood flow to make the penis larger, there has to be no problem with blood flow. For the erection to be sustained, the trapping of this excess blood needs to be efficient. Thus, it all depends upon other factors, so it's complicated. We need to break this down into different areas so that you can see why you have dysfunction in the first place and some of the reasons are explored in the following chapters and will include things such as:

➤ Prostate problems

Prostate health can be a reason for erectile dysfunction. In particular, conditions such as prostate cancer, benign prostatic hyperplasia, hormonal disorders and prostatitis may be responsible for erectile dysfunctions.

When a man's penis suddenly becomes unable to hard up, it may be a symptom of prostate cancer. As such, a doctor may probably require him to take a prostate-specific antigen test or PSA test. The doctor may also require a digital rectal examination to further validate this suspicion.

Prostate cancer surgery runs the risk of severing arteries or nerves that are responsible for a man's erection. Men whose prostate gland has been removed via a surgical procedure called prostatectomy have a 25% to 80% chance of being able to enjoy erections. There are some "nerve-sparing" prostatectomy procedures that try to avoid severing important erectile nerves but even with such methods, erectile dysfunctions have a 50% risk of happening. It's because several factors come into play such as the surgeon's ability, the man's age and the location of the tumor. Even if the key nerves aren't permanently damaged, it'll take anywhere from 6 to 18 months for the nerve fibers to completely regenerate for normal erectile function.

Avoiding surgery to treat prostate cancer can still lead to erectile dysfunctions. Radiation treatment may harm tissues that are vital for experiencing erections. It is estimated that half of the men who underwent radiation treatment for prostate cancer experienced erectile dysfunction due to the external radiation beam as well as the implanted radiation-emitting seeds in the prostate.

Even non-surgical and non-radioactive treatments for cancers that have metastasized beyond the prostate, like some hormone therapy medications, can cause erectile dysfunctions. Some of these medications include goserelin (a.k.a. Zoladex) and leuprolide (a.k.a Lupron). Some hormone-based medications that may cause erectile dysfunction that aren't as bad include bicalutamide (a.k.a. Casodex) and flutamide (a.k.a. Eulexin).

Another medical condition affecting the prostate that can cause erectile dysfunction is benign prostatic hyperplasia or BPH, which is a form of prostate enlargement that isn't cancerous. However, it isn't the condition itself that causes erectile dysfunction but some of the methods used to treat it like the prescription anti-testosterone drug finasteride (a.k.a. Proscar), which has a reported side effect of erectile dysfunction and reduced libido in 3.7% and 3.3% of the men who took it. Alpha-blockers like doxazosin (a.k.a. Cardura), tamsulosin (a.k.a. Flomax) and terazosin (a.k.a. Hyrtrin) are BPH treatment alternatives that have lower risk for erectile dysfunction.

Another prostate condition that can cause erectile dysfunction is prostatitis, which is acute or chronic inflammation of the prostate. Some of the symptoms that may indicate such a condition include frequent and usually painful urination, penile discharges and fever. Severe cases of prostatitis can directly lead to erectile dysfunction while milder ones simply make ejaculation painful, which reduces sexual pleasure and consequently, make it harder to experience normal erection.

➢ Hormones

Sexual interest in a man is largely dependent on testosterone levels in his body. As such, low levels may significantly reduce sexual desire, horniness and eventually, the ability to enjoy erections. Some estimates report that up to 20% of men who suffer erectile dysfunctions have hormonal problems, i.e., hypogonadism or low testosterone levels.

➢ Stress

When a person is stressed out, the body reacts by releasing cortisol and adrenaline. For men, being stressed most of the time can lead to chronically elevated levels of the 2 aforementioned hormones, both of which can cause erectile dysfunction in 2 ways. Indirectly, stress can lead to weakened libido and consequently, less frequent or worse, failure to achieve erections. In a direct manner, the 2 stress hormones can significantly affect blood flow and since erections are all about the flow, it increases the risk of suffering from erectile dysfunctions.

➢ Depression

A man's libido and depression are, unfortunately, tied together. According to Mark Held, PhD, who is a clinical psychologist in Denver, depression changes a person's biochemistry and consequently affects libido. He further notes – and I agree – that it's harder or practically impossible to be horny and depressed at the same time. Further, some medicines taken for managing depression also increase the risk of weakened libido, especially for men.

➤ Self-Worth

A big chunk of experiencing erections has to do with how a person sees himself. The sexier a person feels, the more frequent and longer lasting his erections will be. However, a man who looks lowly upon himself may find it really hard to feel sexy and thus, may have a very difficult time being aroused. As such, erections may come as frequent and as long as rains in the desert and the lines at many supermarkets, respectively.

➤ Substance Abuse

A little alcohol never hurt anyone. In fact, a small amount can help a man feel more relaxed and confident. Too much of it, however, run the risk of negatively affecting the nervous system as well as increase the risk of being fatigued more often, both of which can significantly reduce a man's libido. Some drugs can also plummet your libido such as marijuana, which suppresses testosterone production by inhibiting the pituitary gland.

➤ Sleep

It's hard to get enough sleep these days but that isn't an excuse. Adequate and good quality of sleep is essential for optimal health and mental performance, as well as libido. As with depression, it's practically impossible to be aroused even by the sexiest woman alive when a man is always tired due to lack of sleep. The desire to get enough sleep always trumps the desire to have sex and as such, the sleep card will almost always trump the horniness card and lead to erectile dysfunction.

> Medicines

Most medicines have side effects that vary in kind, duration and intensity. In particular, some medicines used for managing blood pressure, depression and prostate problems increase the risk for erectile dysfunction. Most men who are under medication are aware of this risk on top of others such as drowsiness, dry mouth, headaches, upset stomach and skin irritation, among others. One medication that can cause erectile dysfunction is benzodiazepines – a popular medication for treating anxiety, insomnia and seizures. In particular, popular benzodiazepines like Ativan, Xanax, Librium and Valium have a sedative effect for reducing anxiety. The sedating benefits aren't limited to anxiety however, and often times extend to a man's libido. When the libido is also sedated, it's very challenging to experience frequent and lasting erections.

As mentioned earlier, depression is a sure ball way to quench libido and consequently, keep a man from experiencing erections.

But the treatment for it may not necessarily be the cure – at least for erectile dysfunction. One popular type of antidepressant called selective serotonin reuptake inhibitors (SSRI for brevity) such as Prozac, Celexa, Lexapro and Zoloft are observed to affect about 60% of men who take them. Though there's still no clear reason as to how it does so, it's suspected that erectile dysfunction cases are related to its effect on the neurotransmitter called serotonin, dopamine and norepinephrine. All 3 neurotransmitters affect a person's well-being and as such, can affect libido and ultimately reduce a man's ability to experience erections.

Blood pressure medication – beta-blockers in particular – can also affect a man's ability to achieve and sustain erections. Beta-blockers like Lopressor, SEctral, Tenormin and Cogard can have the same effect on neurotransmitters as antidepressants particularly epinephrine, which affects a man's ability to feel excited. Some studies also suggest that beta-blockers interfere with the part of men's nervous systems responsible for sexual arousal and consequently, erections.

Allergies may have little to do with erectile dysfunction but the medicines used to treat them have much to do with it. Antihistamines like Dramamine and Benadryl were noted to lead to erectile dysfunction, though no clear evidence explains just how they do so. Possibly, it's because it affects the same areas of the nervous system responsible for arousal. The good news is that the erectile dysfunction side effect is temporary and often times disappear soon after stopping such medication.

Medications used to treat digestive system conditions like heartburn, erosive esophagitis, gastric ulcers and acid reflux – also known as H2 blockers – can also lead to erectile dysfunction, especially at high dosages, both indirectly (decreased libido) and directly (erectile dysfunction). H2 blockers also run the risk of reducing a man's sperm count.

> ➤ Other factors which contribute to dysfunction

It's not a time to feel that your masculinity is in question. It's a time to explore to find out why your body is not responding in the way that you expect it to and this is essential to get rid of any doubts you may have and to adjust things so that you have the maximum chances of continuing with a love-life that is satisfying for both of you.

Forget the question of simply finding a solution. It's not the way to approach the problem. The following pages contain very vital information that will give you the right approach to solving the problem forever, so that you can maximize the possibility of overcoming dysfunction and going back to a healthy sex life.

Chapter 4

Erectile Dysfunction Myths

There are many beliefs going on around what causes erectile dysfunctions – some are myths and some are not exactly mythical. So which is which? In this chapter, we'll take a look at some of the most common beliefs about erectile dysfunction and their veracity.

Old = Erectile Dysfunction

Many men believe that one of the reasons for erectile dysfunctions is growing old. Now, it may be true that men's risk for erectile dysfunction increases with age – it is estimated that 4% of men in their 50s, 17% of men in their 60s and 47 of men in their 70s suffer from erectile dysfunction – but that doesn't mean age is the cause of the medical condition. Rather, it's the health problems related to aging that cause erectile dysfunctions such as diabetes, heart problems, testosterone levels and even inflammation.

Simply put, the healthier a man is generally, the higher his chances are of enjoying healthy erections. While men can't stay young forever, they can do something to make sure they stay as healthy – and as virile – as possible even in their golden years.

Tighty whities

Another popular belief running around is that tight underwear can lead to erectile dysfunction. The verdict: it's a myth!

The truth about tighty whities is that it can lead to lower sperm motility, which is a fertility issue and not a potency one. It's because tighty whities or tight underwear can make it too warm for comfort in terms of the testes' ability to produce sperm.

So next time you're feeling scared to put on your Speedoes, just remember it won't keep you from "standing attention".

Too much (self) pleasure kills

Another wildly popular belief is that masturbation leads to erectile dysfunction over time. It doesn't help that if you Google "erectile dysfunction", your search will yield tons of feedback on how much men are worried about "going soft" with too much masturbation.

The verdict: it's a myth! Experts say that to the contrary, masturbation is a sign of a healthy libido (essential for erections) and can potentially help alleviate some kinds of sexual dysfunctions. In fact, masturbation is an encouraged practice for men who are diagnosed with what is known as hypoactive sexual desire and arousal disorders, a.k.a., under-horniness syndrome. Now talk about myths, eh?

One possible reason for the prevalence of such myth is that when it's related to addiction to pornography, which is a valid cause for erectile dysfunction. You'll get to know more about why this is so in a later chapter. But other than that, masturbation can actually help you maintain healthy erections until old age.

Cycling

Lately, riding bicycles have been a concern when it comes to erectile dysfunctions. It's probably due to a study conducted by researchers from the University of California that reported vital arteries and nerves may be affected by this hobby. In particular, hard bike seats can potentially squeeze the area between the scrotum and anus – also known as the perineum – which can lead to significant compression of nerves and arteries necessary for achieving erections.

The verdict: none yet. While the above-mentioned concern is valid, it doesn't take into consideration other biking factors that can cause erectile dysfunction such as the amount of time spent biking, riding style and bike fit. Chances are, the risk for erectile dysfunction is much higher for competitive cyclists who are known to spend more time on their bikes than with their wives.

Just bike in moderation. What is considered moderate? As long as you don't feel pain, numbness and are still able to enjoy erections without difficulty, that's a sign that you're not biking too often and too hard.

Emotional health

Many times, it is believed that erectile dysfunction is psychological or emotional. It is true in some instances. However, a study showed that up to 82% of men with erectile dysfunction also experience depression-like symptoms.

Verdict: In some cases, it's true. The medical community has acknowledged that there are cases wherein the causes of erectile dysfunction is psychological/emotional rather than physiological when it introduced the classification "psychogenic erectile dysfunction" in 2001.

Chapter 5
Are You At Risk?

Is it possible to identify men who are at risk for erectile dysfunction? Some researchers say yes. In particular, there's a method that can reasonably predict who among men receiving prostate cancer treatment are most likely to experience erectile dysfunction due to such treatment. This can be a very helpful tool for helping men decide whether or not to go for prostate cancer treatment immediately or adapt a wait-and-see approach.

In general, prolonging life and increasing the chances of survival are top priorities for treating cancers in general. For prostate cancer, chances of survival are relatively higher compared to others as most men diagnosed with early-stage prostate cancer survive the condition. That being said, another important concern when it comes to treatment are side effects that men may suffer as a result.

Diagnostic tests like the PSA or prostate-specific antigen blood test can reveal tumors in a man's prostate. However, most of these tumors grow at such a tortoise-like pace that they pose very little threat to a man's health. The problem is, such a test only identifies presence of tumors and isn't able to distinguish aggressive ones. As such, most men go for early treatment just to be sure.

These treatments don't come easy – they have side effects too. These may include bowel dysfunction, incontinence and erectile dysfunction, which is the most common side effect. It also happens to be one that most affects men emotionally. As such, any testing procedure that can reasonably predict the chances of men suffering from post-treatment erectile dysfunction can be of great help in making the decision to go for treatment immediately or not.

Dr. Martin Sanda and his colleagues at the Beth Israel Deaconess Medical Center in Boston have developed a test that has an accuracy rate of up to 90% in predicting a man's risk for developing post-treatment erectile dysfunction. According to Dr. Sanda, the test can be administered in a clinical setting and scored within just 7 minutes and that the key is determining a patient's baseline prior to receiving treatment.

Based on their research, they've have suggested that a man's chances of suffering from erectile dysfunction varies based on the kind of prostate cancer treatment administered. They found that men who didn't suffer from erectile dysfunctions prior to receiving prostate cancer treatment had a 60% likelihood of suffering from erectile dysfunction within 2 years after surgical removal of the prostate. They also found that over 40% of men who have never encountered erectile dysfunction and who had received external radiation treatment for prostate cancer experienced erectile dysfunction after the treatment. The figure goes to less than 40% for those who received brachytherapy or had radioactive "seeds" implanted in the prostate.

It was also noted that high PSA levels also increased the risk for post-treatment erectile dysfunction. Race, age, sexual history and body mass index (BMI) were also identified as key pre-treatment variables for assessing one's risk for post-treatment erectile dysfunction together with the type of treatment methods administered.

Restless legs syndrome and erectile dysfunction

Another factor to consider in assessing one's risk for erectile dysfunction is restless legs syndrome. Men who have this, a study suggests, have higher risks for a limp wiener than those who don't.

Restless legs syndrome triggers in a person a strong need to move the legs, particularly because of discomfort when sitting or lying down. Others describe the feeling of restless legs syndrome as a burning, tingling, crawling or creeping sensation and that this sensation seems to diminish when the legs are moved. Such relief, however, is short-lived. Although there are no established causes for this, there are cases that this is caused by pregnancy or anemia and can be aggravated by consuming alcohol, tobacco and caffeine.

This study, conducted by Harvard University researchers, is one that is built on the earlier researches that linked the frequency of erectile dysfunction in men with restless legs syndrome. The study also noted that as the frequency of restless legs syndrome symptoms increase, so do the risk for erectile dysfunction.

The study involved over 11,000 men averaging 64 years of age by the time the trial study started in 2002. Further, these men had no history of erectile dysfunction, arthritis or diabetes. The study started with the men being administered a standard set of health questions. The basis for classifying the men as having restless legs syndrome or RLS is meeting 4 RLS diagnostic criteria and experienced symptoms for more than 5 times monthly.

During the study, 1,979 cases of erectile dysfunction were identified. The study also found that men with RLS had a 50% higher chance of experiencing erectile dysfunction vs. men who didn't have RLS, taking into consideration the subjects' weight, age, and histories for anti-depressants, smoking or chronic diseases. It also noted that men who experienced RLS symptoms by as much as 14 times monthly had a 68% higher chance of struggling with erectile dysfunction.

The 1 January 2010 edition of the Sleep journal also reported that impotence seems to be more prevalent among older men afflicted with restless legs syndrome compared to those that aren't afflicted with RLS and that the higher the frequency of symptoms, the higher were their risks.

Dr. Xiang Gao – who is an instructor at Harvard Medical School – postulated a simple explanation for the link between RLS and impotence. He said that the association between the two may be due to underproduction of dopamine, a brain chemical.

Bradley Martin

Chapter 6

How Porn Can Affect Your Performance

You may be surprised to note that porn can have a devastating effect on your love life. The reasons? These are many but the biggest reason is that porn movies can actually change your perception of what sex should be like and can alter your expectations.

What has been found is that younger and younger men are seeking help for impotence and that his has a direct link to their porn viewing. Sex experts have said that overstimulation of sexual activity is actually something that can and does happen. What this means in terms of performance is that the levels of dopamine in the brain are affected and that this can lead to being unable to sustain an erection.

Porn addiction

Many men are heavily into porn – almost worshipping it like a deity. Why? For one, most men aren't the sexual conquistadors they'd like to be and pornography enables them to fulfill their wildest and biggest sexual fantasies – and more – with all the hottest, nastiest and horniest chicks around. And with the advent of the Internet, it's practically free to indulge in it anytime and anywhere. It's like breathing air for many men!

As with many good things (assuming for the sake of argument that it is "good"), too much of it can be bad. In particular, addiction to the stuff is a very real factor that can contribute to a man's inability to experience erections.

What? Porn addiction can lead to erectile dysfunction? Seriously?

Yes, I'm serious. But before we go further as to how it can lead to erectile dysfunction, let us first find out just how much porn is too much? When does an appetite for beautiful, naked women become an – as one of the popular rock band Guns N' Roses' albums is named – appetite for destruction?

There's a quiz featured in mensfitness.com that was developed by Paula Hall, author of Understanding & Treating Sex Addiction (Routledge, 2012), that can help evaluate whether or not a particular interest in pornography is just "average" or already an addiction. You can – if you wish – take that quiz by answering the following questions, tallying your total scores based on your answer choices and checking it against a grid at the end of the quiz. Just a disclaimer though – this quiz is merely for personal use and shouldn't be used to substitute for a professional assessment and diagnosis.

➤ Do you spend a minimum of 11 hours weekly looking at porn?

Never	=	0
Occasionally	=	1
Often	=	2
Most Of The Time	=	3

➤ Is your relationship with your partner affected negatively by your porn viewing?

Never	=	0
Occasionally	=	1
Often	=	2
Most Of The Time	=	3

➤ Does viewing porn interfere with your work or spending time with friends and family?

Never	=	0
Occasionally	=	1
Often	=	2
Most Of The Time	=	3

➤ Do you prioritize viewing porn over spending time with family and friends?

Never	=	0
Occasionally	=	1
Often	=	2
Most Of The Time	=	3

➤ Do you view porn to relieve boredom or feel happier?

Never	=	0
Occasionally	=	1
Often	=	2
Most Of The Time	=	3

➤ Do you feel that you need to stop viewing porn?

Never   =   0

Occasionally   =   1

Often   =   2

Most Of The Time   =   3

➤ Do you find it challenging to have erections or ejaculate during sex?

Never   =   0

Occasionally   =   1

Often   =   2

Most Of The Time   =   3

➤ Do you have to fantasize about the women you viewed in porn just to get horny for sex?

Never   =   0

Occasionally   =   1

Often   =   2

Most Of The Time   =   3

➤ Do you feel the need to view more and harder-core porn just to maintain the same feelings?

Never	=	0
Occasionally	=	1
Often	=	2
Most Of The Time	=	3

Tally your total score. If you got less than 8 points, you're most likely not addicted to porn – at least not yet. However, if your family has a background of porn addiction, consider yourself to be at risk for becoming an addict. It's highly recommended that you keep your sexual experiences as free from pornography as possible and minimize your dependence on the stuff to manage boredom, stress and sadness. As with some medicines and supplements, your body can develop immunity or resistance to porn, which makes you want to get more and harder-core of it, so intermittent or extended porn fasting can be or great help to minimize your risk for addiction. Doing so helps re-calibrate your body chemical that's responsible for pleasure: dopamine. Think of it as regularly running. The more frequent and farther you run, the more your body becomes tolerant and that when you lay off running for an extended period of time, your body tolerance for it goes down.

If you scored between 9 to 15 points, consider yourself on the cusp of becoming an addict. At this point, you'll need to start taking matters into your own – pardon the pun – hands. Cutting back on your porn viewing is no longer an option – it's a must! This is because pornography can become a poison instead of a medicine that you hope can cure your life's woes away. It's as sensible as trying to get promoted by frequently taking days off from work to sleep at home.

If you scored 16 and above, you can almost – with certainty – dub yourself a porn addict. Chances are, you've attempted to ditch porn for quite a while now but have failed to do so because you're in too deep. As such, self-treatment or self-help is no longer a viable option and it's time to seek help. Consider joining support groups like Sex Addicts Anonymous or get professional help from a qualified therapist.

Too much is too much

As with some of the most enjoyable things in life like alcohol and salty, fatty and sugary foods, masturbation is a very controversial health topic. It's because of the abundance of seemingly scientific but contradicting information on the Internet pertaining to the practice's purported benefits and side effects.

Take for example the health benefits. Studies have reported that masturbation isn't just normal – it's also good for a man's health because it can significantly reduce the risk for prostate problems, help reduce anxiety and consequently, normalize the immune system. On the other hand, there are also reports of excessive masturbation causing more frequent cases of erectile dysfunction among men.

Honestly, those aren't contradictory. It's a well-established fact that too much of good things can ultimately cause harm. Protein is good for the body but if you eat too much of it, especially if you have kidney problems already, you run the risk of renal failure. Lifting weights at the gym is definitely beneficial in terms of building physical strength but lifting too much weight and too frequently – i.e., not enough rest – can lead to injuries like muscle and joint tears. And just like Brian May – he of the famous rock band Queen – wrote and sang, too much love can kill you.

When a man becomes addicted to porn, his view of females alters as well. He sees all women as potential porn stars, which of course they are. They participate in sexual acts and although they don't do this behind a camera, they could. Thus, men who are addicted to Internet porn are unlikely to distinguish between their partner and the women that they see on the screen. The reality, of course, is much different. His expectations of his partner become exaggerated.

Another thing about porn and masturbation addiction is that it can cause a man to be more anxious about his sexual performance. He'll start to believe that the "passing grade" for sexual performance is the ones he sees on porn – inhumanly large penises, mutant abilities to hold off ejaculation despite all the nasty and horny stuff women do to those well-endowed sex-marathon men. Because he starts to believe that such superhuman characteristics are the standards, he'll feel so inadequate and will start to see himself as unworthy, leading to low self-worth. And as mentioned in an earlier chapter, a man who looks lowly upon himself will have a hard time feeling aroused and may struggle to experience erections.

It also affects an area of the brain called the frontal cortex. This part of the brain is used for sending messages to the body and planning action. Thus, if over or under stimulated, it appears that the frontal cortex messages can become distorted and impotence may result. The messages needed from the brain to the penis are not getting through clearly and thus it's impossible to become erect.

Scientists found through study of a case where a man had sustained serious damage to this area of the brain that this frontal cortex also determines the kind of person that someone is. A damaged frontal cortex was responsible for changes in behavior by one man, who, unfortunately, suffered an accident which pierced the area in question. Although he survived, he was not able to continue to be the mild and polite man that he was before the accident.

Another reason why excess of porn or porn addition can alter a man's perception of what lovemaking should be is that it stimulates unhealthy interest in porn, rather than realistic lovemaking and closes off the mind to anything other than that as being normal. Thus, he becomes disinterested in normal stimuli and can rely upon porn rather than **real** sex as something that satisfied his sexual needs. Thus, with this very unrealistic view of sex, a man may not achieve erection because the picture in his brain of raw porn sex is more interesting and vital to the man than real sex ever can be.

With over stimulation of the frontal cortex, this area begins to erode, so that the personality of the man is affected as well.

Too much masturbation is also considered an addiction – one that's exacerbated by pornography. When experiencing any pleasurable stimuli, e.g., food or sex, the body releases dopamine, which is considered the "pleasure" chemical. When men watch porn and masturbate, there's a flood of dopamine going around the system. Doing this frequently makes the receptors responsible for generating feelings of sexual pleasure and arousal more and more conditioned to dopamine – making it less and less sensitive over time. When this happens, the same sexual stimuli becomes less potent and over time is rendered useless in terms of sexual arousal and erection. More – in terms of frequency and intensity – sexual stimuli is required to reach the same sexual arousal and erection and becomes a downward spiral of decreasing libido and erections. At this point, a man starts to suffer erectile dysfunction.

If you're at that stage already, what's the solution? Simple – stop viewing porn and masturbating. Go on long porn and masturbation fast – ideally about 12 weeks. This is to reacclimatize your brain and your psyche to normal human sex standards and reset your libido to make it healthy and help you achieve regular and healthy erections again.

The bottom line

If you have begun to use porn as a stimuli and it's more important than real life, then you need help. Even though your love life may not be initially affected by what you watch, the eventual breakdown of different elements of your love life is inevitable and that includes becoming impotent.

If you have experienced the inability to have an erection or sustain one and are always looking for the next opportunity to watch porn, then you need to see someone who can help you to train this addiction so that it does not change the person that you are or affect your ability to make love in a normal way with a healthy erection that will stay the course.

Chapter 7

External Influences That Affect Your Sex Life

There are several factors that affect how you get an erection and whether you can sustain it. Some of these are things that you need to personally address because they could be affecting the way that you perform.

Alcohol, Tobacco and Substance Abuse

As mentioned earlier, substance abuse, i.e., drugs, alcohol and nicotine can significantly increase a man's risk for erectile dysfunction and is often times an offshoot of poor stress management – people run to these substances to release stress. And unfortunately, these substances contribute to the very essence of erectile dysfunction – poor blood circulation, especially in the penis.

Let's take a look at smoking first. Studies have shown that the main harmful ingredient in cigarette smoking – nicotine – leads to constricted blood vessels and in particular, increases one's risk for atherosclerosis wherein the arteries harden. Nicotine does this by inhibiting the body's ability to produce nitric oxide, a substance that helps improve blood flow. Smoking leads to less available nitric oxide in the arteries, which leads to poor blood circulation. And that is one sure way to kill erection. If there's a best time to quit smoking, it is now.

Let's now look at alcoholic drinks. For most people, substance abuse merely pertains to drugs and doesn't count alcohol as a deadly substance particularly if consumption is at most, moderate. Part of the belief is the result of studies that show occasional alcohol consumption – red wine in particular – has healthy benefits both physical and emotional.

Speaking of emotional benefits, drinking alcohol helps people feel more positive. It's because alcohol can act as some kind of anti-depressant – helping shut down the negative-talk monster inside the mind for a period of time. As such, it helps people feel happier, more confident and to some extent – hornier.

You may be surprised to learn that despite suppressing sexual inhibitions for the moment, drinking alcohol can still cause men to suffer from a flaccid penis also known as "brewers' droop".

Although this effect is just temporary, it can ruin a man's sexual plans for the night when he finds that however horny he feels, his "mini-me" isn't up to the task.

Over the long term, alcoholism can seriously affect a man's ability to experience erections, i.e. chronic erectile dysfunction. It's because heavy consumption of alcohol for extended periods of time, e.g., alcoholism, can lead to damaged nerves. In particular, it can lead to permanent damage in the nerves that connect both man's heads, i.e., the brain and the penis. Permanent erectile dysfunction due to alcoholism is also known as alcohol-induced impotence.

Apart from nerve damage, alcoholism also leads to erectile dysfunction by affecting a man's hormones particularly testosterone, which you learned in an earlier chapter to be crucial for having enough libido to experience erections. At this point, it is well worth evaluating the pleasures brought about by drinking alcohol and sexual pleasures and to choose wisely between the two. Just bear in mind that moderate drinking is probably ok but it's best to avoid drinking altogether if you want to minimize your risk for erectile dysfunction.

Lastly, let's talk about drugs and how they significantly increase the risk for erectile dysfunction. There are two kinds: psychoactive and prescription ones. Psychoactive drugs such as barbiturates, amphetamines, marijuana, cocaine, opiates and methadone can cause erectile dysfunction in 2 ways: central nervous system and blood circulation. Avoid these unless prescribed by your doctor and talk to him or her as soon as you notice that using such is interfering with your ability to experience erections.

Prescription drugs can also be abused, though not necessarily on a recreational level. As mentioned earlier, blood pressure medications, anti-depressants, sedatives and tranquilizers can increase your risk for erectile dysfunction.

Obesity

One demographic that's at very high risk for erectile dysfunction are men who are obese. Yes, there are many other factors responsible for erectile dysfunction but even an emotionally and physically healthy man can still fall prey to this condition if he is overweight. The connection between being overweight and the ability to experience erections is a strong one and it is estimated that on average, the risk of suffering from erectile dysfunction is 2.5 times higher for obese men than those who weigh normally.

But what is obesity, really? How can we objectively classify a person as obese or not? There are several ways to do it that are beyond the scope of this e-book but all of those methods have one thing in common: they have established benchmarks of what is considered to be healthy weight based on a person's height and age, among other things.

So how does being obese keep a man from experiencing erections? Do you still remember what makes for an erection? Yes, blood flow to the penis is what makes erections possible. Obesity increases a person's risk for atherosclerosis or constricted arteries due to accumulated cholesterol on the blood vessels' walls. The tighter the arteries are, the less blood flows to the organs, which includes a man's penis.

Another way obesity can keep a man from experiencing erections is by reducing the amount of testosterone. As you have learned earlier, testosterone plays a huge part in feeling aroused and eventually, having erections. In particular, testosterone increases the nitric oxide and this substance helps increase blood flow to the penis.

Obesity is the single biggest risk factor for cardiovascular disease and since sexual and cardiovascular health are closely related, erectile dysfunction can – in some cases – be a symptom of heart problems in obese men. Researchers from a leading university in Italy found that men who were diagnosed to have heart problems started to experience erectile dysfunction as early as 2 to 3 years prior. Doctors at a leading university in the United States also found that erectile dysfunction can be an indicator or warning sign of future strokes and heart problems.

Obesity doesn't just physically affect a man's ability to experience erections – it also does so psychologically. Because obesity can lead to significantly lower testosterone levels, obese men are vulnerable to experiencing low libido, feeling depressed and having low energy. Synergistically, these can kill a man's hope for a satisfying sex life and lead to or exacerbate existing erectile problems.

Fortunately, obesity isn't as complicated to address. With the right amount and types of exercises coupled with a sound nutrition plan, losing excess weight is highly achievable and safe. A leading center in Italy noted that 1/3 of obese men who lost significant weight reported better sexual functions afterwards.

Weight loss, especially huge ones, can look daunting at first but it isn't. What makes it so is the pressure to lose a lot of the excess pounds asap, which isn't just unrealistic but also unhealthy in the long run. Healthy weight loss is at most 2 pounds a week – cutting just 500 to 1,000 calories daily. Losing more than 2 pounds weekly run the risk of losing more water and muscles mass instead of fat. Fewer muscles mean a slower metabolism and consequently less ability to burn calories and fat.

When trying to lose fat, it's important to monitor food consumption, particularly the kinds of calories and the amount of calories. Some of the best guidelines to follow for a successful and sustainable weight loss include:

-Know your average daily caloric requirements for maintaining your current weight.

-Don't cut daily calories by more than 15% and don't do it for more than 4 days straight. Every 5th day, bump up consumption to 10% more than your maintenance in order to "trick" your body into believing there's enough calories going around and prevent it from slowing down metabolism as a survival instinct. Extended crash diets lead to weight loss plateaus because such practices tell the body that calories are scarce, making it slow down metabolism to survive.

-Stick with good carbohydrates like oats, brown rice, whole wheat breads, fruits and vegetables. Avoid sugary foods and drinks as well as processed carbohydrates like white bread. They can wreak havoc on your energy levels and metabolism.

-Increase your protein intake. Apart from extending feelings of being full, protein helps build and maintain muscle mass, which is crucial for maintaining a healthy metabolism.

-Eat whole foods instead of processed ones. As a rule of thumb, courtesy of the Paleo diet people, the more a food item resembles its original form, the healthier it is. For example, roasted chicken (you can tell that it is chicken) is definitely healthier than chicken nuggets (really, how can you be sure they're made from chicken, eh?).

-Limit your consumption of oil-fried food. Even if you use canola and olive oils (healthy oils), heating them past a certain point alters their molecular structure and strips them of their healthiness.

The other half of the successful weight loss equation is exercise. Apart from weight loss, it has been reported that men who are physically active with exercise have a 30% lower risk for erectile dysfunction than those who just exercise mentally. Here are a couple of helpful exercise guidelines for successful weight loss:

-Take baby steps. Don't expect to immediately run 10 kilometers straight if you can't even walk 2 kilometers without stopping. Gradually build up your capacity to avoid burning out or worse, getting injured.

-Don't baby it too much too. You need to exercise at an intensity that's challenging enough it burns calories. If you're used to walking 1 kilometer straight comfortably, aim for 1.5

kilometers the next time and when you become comfortable with that already, go for 2 kilometers and so on. The point is don't baby yourself.

-The right intensity is key. There are several, high-tech ways of determining the intensity level but of course, those are too much of a hassle and are expensive. Just use the talk test to find out. While exercising, try talking. If you're able to comfortably carry a normal conversation while doing so, you're exercise intensity is too light. If you're barely able to say a word, it's too intense. If you're still able to carry a normal conversation although with some difficulty, that's moderately intense. Go for moderate intensity, which is optimal for long-term weight loss success.

-Exercise continuously at moderate intensity for at least 20 minutes for at least 3 times a week for best results.

-If you're hitting the gym to lift weights, it's best to let at least 48 hours pass before working out the same muscle group again. Muscles need 48 hours to fully recuperate before being worked out again with resistance exercises such as weight lifting.

-Don't force it. If you're feeling some pain or are sick, skip the exercise session for that day. You'll just make things worse if you push through.

Mental

Although erectile dysfunction is mostly a physiological problem, psychogenic causes can also account for it or even exacerbate the situation. As you learned earlier, stress, anxiety and depression can affect a man's ability to be aroused and the medications used for treating psychogenic causes also have the same effect. Psychogenic causes of erectile dysfunction may include the following:

-Depression;

-Dysfunctional view of sex;

-Marriage problems;

-Sexual performance worries;

-Previous sexual traumas;

-Personal beliefs and inhibitions; and

-Sex phobias.

Psychological erectile dysfunction can be caused by persisting psychological issues like chronic depression, obsessive-compulsive disorder (OCD), manic depression, general anxiety disorder (GAD), schizophrenia, post-traumatic stress disorder, borderline personality disorder, attention deficit- hyperactivity disorder and unresolved personal issues. The good news is most men's erectile dysfunctions aren't caused by major psychogenic causes nor do such men share a common profile according to a study by Weeks and Gambescia in 2000.

Erectile dysfunctions caused by temporary mental difficulties like depression or anxiety brought about by major events like job loss or death of a family member are called psychological distress erectile dysfunction. It is believed that almost half of the population may experience such major events at least once in their lives and as such, puts many men at risk for such an erectile dysfunction. In many cases, it can be challenging to determine which causes which, the erectile dysfunction or the mental difficulty. The good news is that this kind of erectile dysfunction is often intermittent in nature and as such, isn't chronic and can be easily addressed.

Psychological stress is often underestimated by men when it comes to sexual potency and as such, often attribute their inability to achieve erections to heavier, more profound reasons. Truth is, it only takes some form of psychological stress to interfere with normal sexual functioning and experiencing erectile dysfunction is highly likelier when he experiences reactive depression, situational anxiety, self doubt, lack of confidence, irritation, disappointment, embarrassment, remorse, unrealistic sexual expectations about himself and personal conflicts.

Erectile dysfunction can also occur due to lack of necessary behavioral, emotional and cognitive sexual abilities for successful and pleasurable lovemaking. In other words, a man's lack of confidence in terms of his looks, his penile size and his ability to please his lover can cause him to lose hope and interest in sex and can lead to his penis' inability to "stand up and take notice". The thing with this kind of erectile dysfunction is that unless the psychological issue is addressed, it can persist for life. However, this kind of dysfunction is limited to actual lovemaking alone. A man who suffers from this kind of erectile dysfunction can still have erections when masturbating alone because in such a situation, he's in full control and thus feels relaxed, comfortable and confident, which allows him to be aroused and experience erections.

So how can psychological erectile dysfunctions be addressed? One way is through what is known as the Cognitive-Behavioral-Emotional model, also known as the CBE model. This particular model acknowledges that each man is made up of thoughts (cognition), actions (behavior) and feelings (emotions), which comprise the core of what needs to be addressed in dealing with psychological erectile dysfunction. Let's first consider thoughts or cognitions.

Thoughts or cognitions are made up of a person's beliefs, ideas, observations, assumptions, expectations, interpretations and perceptions. They can either be good or bad for the person, depending on their effect on the person and the way that person feels and acts. Thoughts are the major drivers of one's emotions and a persons thoughts about key sexual issues, e.g., standards for lovemaking, sexual beliefs, assumptions, expectations and perceptions about sex in general and about himself in particular, are keys to how he can perform and feel satisfied sexually. As such, it is crucial that one's sexual thoughts are well grounded on realistic and reasonable ideas about one's sexual relationship, ability to respond sexually and one's body. It's important to be able to think positive and realistic sexual thoughts instead of negative and unrealistic ones.

Now let's talk about actions or behaviors, which are dependent on our thoughts and emotions. One of the most prevalent myths about behavior is that it's a reaction. No it isn't. At the end of the day, behavior or actions are decisions made by an individual. If a person withdraws from any opportunity for sexual contact because of feelings of insecurity, it's a decision made by the individual to let such feelings rule and to withdraw. Without his consent, withdrawal from such opportunities won't be possible. Responsible and accountable men exercise control over their actions or behavior and don't let their feelings rule them. It's worth noting that in many cases, feelings and thoughts can be influenced by – you guessed it right – actions or behavior.

Now let's discuss feelings or emotions. These may be considered as electrical and chemical events that the body experiences and are labeled accordingly per physical sensation experienced like sadness, fear, dread, loneliness, resentment, satisfaction, contentment, worry, pleasure, frustration, excitement, irritability, surprise, anxiety, shame, confusion, comfort, embarrassment and guilt. Feelings or emotions motivate people to act or respond to actions either by rewarding or penalizing such. These aren't inherently right or wrong, good or bad – only how we handle them. Feelings or emotions can influence the way we think (thoughts or cognitions) as well as our behaviors (actions). Proper emotional management is key to successfully overcome psychological erectile dysfunction.

The 3 aforementioned components – thoughts, behaviors and feelings – can have numerous and complicated interactions or relationships. Our thoughts can help shape our feelings, feelings can mold thoughts, feelings and thoughts can cause us to behave in different ways and consistent behavior or actions can also help shape the way we think and feel. For example, if we (men) think that we won't get an erection, we can either feel discouraged (feelings), un-aroused (feelings) and ultimately avoid any opportunities for sexual contact (actions), which can further reinforce the feelings and thoughts that prompted it. Another example would be that despite feeling inadequate (feelings), we can choose to take the risk of initiating and experiencing sexual contact (behavior) and discover that what we felt wasn't accurate (thoughts) and actually feel good about ourselves afterwards (feelings) enough to do it again in the future (behavior).

This is the heart of the CBE model: to recognize how behaviors, feelings and thoughts influence each other and actively manage them to achieve lasting desired change, e.g., address psychological erectile dysfunction.

Relationships

Relationship issues can also be factors that lead to erectile dysfunctions among men. One of them is relationship distress caused by complicated dynamics at work in a man's relationships, e.g., communications failures, infidelity issues and conflicts. It may also be possible that this is a result of ED.

Using the aforementioned CBE model, the focus is on 3 critical dimensions of satisfactory intimate relationships: identity, cooperation and intimacy. Let's look at identity first.

Relationship identity refers to general thoughts about the relationship, e.g., expectations, beliefs and attributions that each partner brings into it. It also includes, among others, each partner's personal history and how the relationship means to each. One good example is the issue of how much individual freedom each partner needs to keep the relationship going strong. Some individuals – usually men – require a great degree of autonomy and may despise having to need the other partner's consent to be able to do some of the things he enjoys like playing golf or going out for a round of drinks with the guys. Healthy intimate relationships benefit each partner enough that they bring in beneficial attributes to the same relationship, creating an upward spiral of intimate relationship.

Now let's consider the role of cooperation in maintaining healthy and intimate relationships. Relationship cooperation refers to how each partners overall behavioral interactions within the relationship, e.g., how they work together, how they communicate and how they resolve conflicts. Each partner's thoughts and feelings, unless communicated, remain hidden. In particular, negative sexual thoughts and feelings that are unexpressed remain unresolved and can significantly affect a couple's sexual relationship and can be a factor in the man's ability to have erections.

Lastly, let's discuss intimacy. This refers to a relationships overall climate or level of emotional connection and includes sex, friendship and emotions and are generally characterized by feelings of closeness, commitment and affections. Without a deep level of intimacy, relationships will be shallow. Eventually, shallow relationships become less and less conducive for a healthy sexual one and can contribute to erectile dysfunction for men.

The same principle applied in the CBE model can also be used to address relationship distress erectile dysfunction: knowing how intimacy, cooperation and identity work together allows a man to enhance the quality of his sexual relationship with his partner and in doing so, reduces the incidences of relationship distress and consequently, the risk or incidence of erectile dysfunction.

Where to go from here

A visit to the doctor is essential. Yes, it's embarrassing telling a doctor that you cannot do what most men take for granted. Let's explain why it's so hard (pun intended!).

The male psyche is that of the "doer" and thus, when you find that you can't do something, it frustrates you and there are battles inside you because you feel you should be able to do this. The male is quite upset by the fact that something isn't working that should, and may experience denial for a while because it is too sensitive to discuss.

However, what a man needs to know is that a woman thinks of these things in a totally different manner. She doesn't apportion blame. If anything, she may feel that she isn't doing enough to help her man and will be only too happy to talk with the doctor and her man to help him to overcome whatever the cause may be. She is his best ally when approaching the doctor, and can come up with observations that a man may be too embarrassed to talk about. The female psyche is tuned to the emotional side of the relationship, and she will care sufficiently to want to help. It's her nature.

When you go to the doctor, there are likely to be all kinds of questions. He may ask for blood tests or urine examinations to eliminate certain causes. He may also see external reasons why your sex life isn't happening such as those mentioned above, and may be able to help you in your attempts to overcome problems which you can do something about.

Adjustments to Your Medical Regime

The doctor will also be able to do blood tests that will help him to establish if you are having this problem because of medical reasons. Perhaps the drugs that you take are those which affect whether you can sustain an erection. There are many drugs which do affect the sexual organs and you need to eliminate these as a possibility. If medicine is found to be the cause, there may be alternative medicines less known to affect your sex life as one of the side effects of taking that medication. Therefore, your visit to the doctor should include explaining to him exactly what medications you have been taking.

He may also ask when the problem started and other personal questions, and having your partner there with you will help to give him a fuller picture of what is happening.

Don't expect Viagra as an option straight away

Your body may not need drugs to help you to sustain an erection. There may be other reasons behind the dysfunction, and taking Viagra is not advised for everyone because of other complications that are associated with this drug. Never buy this drug online, believing that it will be the answer to your problems. You need to see a doctor and discuss all of the implications, as well as having a full record of your current health situation, which online suppliers will not have.

Whatever the problem is, it's taken a while to happen. This may be because of clogged blood vessels, it may be because you have stresses and worries, it may be because you are obese or on stimulants such as cigarettes or are drinking too much coffee or alcohol, but it may also be because there is a lack of dialog between your partner and yourself, and that's really one of the most important aspects that you need to explore.

Bradley Martin

Chapter 8
Dialog with Your Partner

If you find that you are not stimulated sufficiently to sustain an erection, it may not be your fault. It may be that you haven't discovered those triggers that help you to maintain your erection. Talking about your sex life with your partner is a great idea. You may not see it as a great idea at this moment in time. You may feel that you are failing her, or that you have some kind of defect. The problem with being a male is that you expect things to happen and in this particular case, they didn't.

Choose a time when you can sit down and talk to your partner. If she sees that you are worried, she will be open to dialog. Don't apportion any blame at all, because even if she isn't that enthused about sex, it's worked until now. Now that the problem has happened, changes need to be made to try to find solutions between the two of you. See how open she is to helping. You may find that your partner is much more open than you think.

Sometimes sustaining an erection depends upon the stimulation of the penis and the sexual position. There are some positions which give the penis more stimulation than others. Talk about fantasies. Talk about the area of the penis which is most sensitive and let her experience playing with this part of your anatomy. It's a great turn on to talk to her about her trigger points as well, so that this isn't just about you. Perhaps you have been through rough times together and you may well be taking these worries to bed with you. It's time to learn to switch off at bedtime and concentrate on the things that matter in that moment in time.

One particularly good sexual position to help a man to stay firm and erect is a deep thrust position commonly known as doggy fashion. The reason for this is because the woman can adjust her position to give more friction and it is this friction that helps the penis to stay erect. This position is where the woman kneels and leans forward and the male approaches her from behind. This would follow foreplay and is a very good position for those whose erection seems half-hearted, for whatever reason. It helps the man to be able to ejaculate and it also helps the woman to gain a great deal of satisfaction because of the depth of the thrust.

There may be things that you haven't discussed with your partner that are making your sex life impossible. For example, prolonged periods of no sexual activity may make it harder for you to trigger those feelings of sexuality. It this is the case, learn to explore each other's bodies and learn what those triggers are. If they are never explored, how can you expect them to go off at the right time? Be caring and try to help your partner to discuss her fantasies. Perhaps the reason why you are experiencing dysfunction is because there isn't enough stimulation between you. If you don't have foreplay, she is likely to be less receptive or drier, especially if over 60. The menopause may be what is putting her off having sex and this rejection of your advances may be contributing to your inability to sustain an erection. In this case, there are lubricants that you can discreetly use to make the possibility of sex better for both of you.

Many people recoil. They don't discuss their fears. They don't discuss their weaknesses, and even if the dysfunction is temporary and a side effect of something else, those men who do not enter into dialog with their women may never discover the cause of that dysfunction, and both partners may be equally frustrated by the dysfunction that is happening. Let it be a prompt for discussion, so that mutual understanding of all your trigger points and hers can open up new feelings that may bring back the ability to make love without the need for medical help.

Remember that there are a certain amount of things that you have under your control that can aid you. Cut out the drink. Cut down on the smoking and try to keep relatively fit. People who are too tired at night may not think sexual thoughts but prefer to simply go to sleep. If you exercise regularly and keep yourself in good shape, then this can come back permanently and your love life can be revived simply by taking action and doing something positive to help restore the body flow and its fitness levels.

This isn't the end of the road. Of course there are medical options, but the first stop should be talking with your partner to try and improve things between you, to try and calm your fears and enlist her help in overcoming your problems. You may be very surprised at how differently you feel about making love, when your partner listens to your needs and is able to make love with you, rather than simply being there. Sex therapists teach people methods that they can learn themselves by exploring each other's bodies and allowing for the fact that life's bumpy road occasionally gets in the way of great sex.

Chapter 9
Medical Possibilities

The doctor needs to know your background if all else has failed, but it's never the end of the line. Don't give up on trying to find out what is happening to your body. There may be reasons for your dysfunction that can be easily remedied. A change of medication, for example, may be all that is required. He will test different things to establish if you have an illness of any kind which may be affecting your ability to stay or to get erect. The percentage of people who suffer from erectile dysfunction due to medical reasons is high at 85 percent, so you shouldn't feel too badly about your situation. It is only 15 percent of cases where psychological problems may be kicking in. Thus, if talking to your partner and trying different things didn't work, it's not the end of the search.

With fifty percent of cases of erectile dysfunction being put down to high blood pressure, this actually makes the problem more manageable if you tackle the reasons for the high blood pressure. The easy way is to take medication, but that doesn't help you long term. It's better to tackle the problem from a more permanent stance. Diabetes and cardio vascular diseases make up the other proportion of reasons for sexual impotence but again treatments are available that may turn the whole situation around. You need to accept responsibility for your body and that means looking after your heart, your blood pressure and the possibility of diabetes and heart disease and listening carefully to the advice given by doctors.

Exercise and a change of diet and lifestyle can really turn things around, and doctors can give you all the right encouragement and advice on how to maximize your recovery times. For example, don't just do certain exercises because you think they will improve a set medical condition. Listen to experts because you may be doing exercises that aggravate the situation rather than making it better. Talk to nutritionists about the changes you need to make in your food intake.

Understand the food triangle and begin to eat healthy portions of food. Although you may have become accustomed to living in a certain way, that way of life may be exactly what led you here looking for answers. Ask your doctor what you can do to get back to a level of fitness that will help you to be able to make love again.

Your body is telling you there is a problem. You can fix it and restore your love life and go on to having very healthy sex.

Pills and potions

It may be that your blood pressure level is something that can be controlled by pills. However, be aware that your lifestyle may also help you to control your blood pressure and to reduce the treatments that you currently take. If you are not overweight, but your blood pressure is high, a doctor may simply prescribe drugs which help you to bring the blood pressure level down and normalize things. Do make the doctor aware of your difficulties with sustaining an erection so that he avoids giving you any medication which may have side effects which inhibit sexual response.

Gadgets and devices

Until you have sorted out your problems with getting an erection, you can try out a vacuum device but if you opt for this, this is a temporary solution to help you to get through that period of obesity or sexual dysfunction. It isn't a permanent solution but something that can make you feel better about yourself and your performance while you tackle the long-term problems which have made you unable to sustain an erection. This way, your partner and you will be able to have a great sex life, but you will also be able to continue your exercise and lifestyle change so that long term, your natural ability to retain an erection will return.

The vacuum pump works in that it helps your penis to retain the blood needed to have an erection. In the case of those who cannot sustain erection, the blood flow is not stemmed and this is vital to retaining erection. A device is used and this has a pump that gets you erect within a very short space of time. Some pumps are one handed while others require two hands, but there's no reason why you can't share the experience with your partner and make it part of your sexual rapport until you get your lifestyle at a level when all of this happens naturally. A ring is placed at the base of the penis to cnsure that the blood within the penis stays in place so that the erection is sufficient to please both you and your partner.

Shock therapy

Researchers have found another treatment method that may spell the doom of drugs like Viagra, Cialis or Levitra: shock therapy. That's right, low-intensity shock therapy on a man's love stick has the potential to be a more effective erectile dysfunction treatment for men suffering from severe cases of the condition.

I know, it gives the impression of a painful experience where electricity is jolted onto the penis head, sending the poor shmuck into a state of intense pain and shock. No, that's not the way it goes. This therapy simply sends through the man's body low-level waves of sound and this kind of treatment has been used to treat tendonitis and plantar fasciitis and similarly, to break up kidney stones via a treatment called lithotripsy.

A study that came out in the Journal of Sexual Health revealed that 34% of the subject men – who responded poorly to oral medications for erectile dysfunction such as Viagra – regained full sexual function after the treatment without taking any medication. It also revealed that all 29 men subjects of the study had an improved response to the drug after the treatment.

Pelvic exercises

There are specific exercises geared to strengthening your pelvic floor, and this helps considerably in being able to retain an erection. In these exercises, you simply lie on your back with your legs folded and your knees together. Imagine the area of your scrotum and with your hands on the front of your hips, pull this area upward. That doesn't mean lifting your body from the mat. It means pulling just that pelvic floor area. This exercise can be done with your legs together or with your legs apart and is far more effective with the knees together.

It's worthwhile investigating exercises that will help to strengthen the pelvic region and these include muscle strengthening of the pelvic basin as well as the area within your shorts. Ask your doctor for a fact sheet on these exercises as these are very good to help you through that dry patch when you are suffering from sexual dysfunction. It takes time to get your body back to its natural state of health and in the meantime, these exercises can help you move forward.

Remember that sexual dysfunction can be caused because you expect it to happen. This is extremely important. If a man has performed badly in bed, it hurts him psychologically because he cannot perform the role that he expects himself to perform. Erection may be achieved and then lost when stopping to put on a condom, for example. He may not be able to sustain the erection, but that failure will play highly on his mind the next time that he makes love. He will fear that failure and that fear can make the failure more likely. If this is the case, then it may be useful to visit a sexologist who can discuss what happens at each stage and reassure him of ways that he can overcome these problems.

It's a huge blow to the male psyche to realize that he cannot perform what he sees as his masculine role. One could even compare this with a woman being told she will never have children. It hurts. Expect it to, and if your dysfunction is caused initially by something going wrong and then continues because of that fear of failure, the best way forward is to talk to a specialist in this field of medicine who will be able to talk you through the problems that are being experienced, and help you to gain confidence again so that your love life is not impacted by erectile dysfunction. Go with your partner. Listen to what the specialist says. His experience will help you through this period and help you toward a much more rewarding sexual experience in the future.

Sexual impotence isn't just something that old people suffer from. It can be a real problem for younger men as well. Perhaps they are concentrating too much of their effort on other things and sexual issues arise because the body needs toning up and training in the right direction. Impotence does happen in old age, but today men are able to continue with a great love life because there are aids available and medicine to help them to retain that close contact with their partners that they desire. Take advantage of this by learning through professionals, and your love life will spring back to life again and you will experience the possibilities open to you through your health provider.

Bradley Martin

Chapter 10

Exercise To Help Erectile Dysfunction

As mentioned earlier, there are specific pelvic floor exercises which can help to deal with erectile dysfunction. However, recent research suggests that ordinary run of the mill exercise can also help. Just walking for half an hour, a few times a week can actually help with erectile dysfunction, because it boosts the circulation, and that's important, because to achieve and sustain an erection, you need good blood flow into the penis. Anything that helps the general circulation in the body will also help with that.

Here's the science bit. What helps the penis to become and remain erect is the health of the endothelium. That's the inner lining of the blood vessels, and it's a big aid to helping the blood flow smoothly and efficiently through the body. Regular exercise is known to maintain the health of the endothelium and thus keep the circulation at a healthy level. That means if you exercise regularly, not only will you keep your heart healthy, you could solve your erection problems at the same time.

There's good news here for the older guys too. Although erectile dysfunction can be a common problem of old age, regular exercise can hold back the aging process by counteracting the natural effects of aging on the blood vessels, and with it, the risk of problems in the bedroom in later life.

It doesn't have to mean pounding the streets or sweating it out in the gym either – walking and swimming are aerobic exercises which can help to keep the endothelium healthy and thus improve the circulation and enhance blood flow to the penis. Studies suggest that walking for 30 minutes a day can reduce the risk of developing erectile dysfunction by around 41%, so it's worth a try. It's also important to do something you enjoy in the way of exercise, because that way, you're more likely to stick with it. Almost said keep it up there, but maybe that's a pun too far!

Experts advise against cycling if you have potency problems, since it can cause damage to the nerves responsible for erections. However, it's okay to use an exercise cycle at home or in the gym, as the seat is likely to be wider and more comfortable than a conventional cycle saddle. Therefore the risk of nerve damage is significantly reduced.

Exercise releases 'feel good' endorphins in the body, and that helps to combat stress and depression. Stress is very often a cause or a contributory factor in erectile dysfunction, and so is depression, and regular exercise can help tackle that. Also, if you need to lose a little weight and build muscle definition to give your self-esteem a boost, exercise can do that too. That's not to say that exercise is the answer to all your problems, but it can certainly help with them, and when you remember that exercise helps to lower blood pressure and stabilize blood glucose levels, you're taking a giant step towards good health, by preventing or treating hypertension and diabetes.

Another benefit of exercise is that it helps you to sleep well, so your body has time to do all the repairs it needs to do to keep you healthy. Lack of sleep can lead to fatigue during the day, and this can interfere with your ability to achieve and maintain an erection. And of course, lack of sleep can lead to stress and even heart disease, so as well as helping with your potency problems, exercise can also help you to stay generally healthy.

Exercise helps you to get slim and stay slim, and as well as improving your self-esteem and confidence, it could help you to avoid or overcome erectile dysfunction. Research suggests that a man with a 32"waist is 50% less likely to have problems with sexual performance than a man with a 42" waist, so there really is something in this exercise lark.

Kegel exercises

As has been mentioned before, there are certain pelvic floor exercises that men can do to help overcome erectile dysfunction. Also known as pelvic floor exercises, they are simple to perform, and can also help guard against other men's health problems such as urinary incontinence and prostate problems.

One really effective trick is to halt the flow of urine midstream several times. This identifies the muscles that need to be used in the Kegel exercises, because unless you identify and locate the right set of muscles, you won't gain any benefits from the exercises. To do the exercise, squeeze the muscles, hold the pose for a count of 5, then release. Repeat this 10 – 20 times, three times a day. The exercise can be done in any position, but it's a good idea to ring the changes and do them standing up, sitting down or lying down. That makes sure all the muscles are used.

Another good Kegel is to clench the muscles of the anus, as if you're trying to stop yourself from going to the toilet. Hold it for between 5 and 10 seconds, then release. Repeat 10 times. When you're doing Kegels, remember to keep breathing naturally. Don't hold your breath, because that will deprive the muscles of the oxygen they need to function properly. And just use the muscles you isolated and identified – resist the temptation to use muscles in your stomach, buttocks or thighs – that won't do you any favors at all.

Because these exercises strengthen the pelvic floor muscles and increase blood supply to the penis, they also have the potential to allow you to enjoy even better orgasms, since performing Kegels regularly enhances sexual sensation. This is partly because you become more in tune with your body as a result of isolating and working the pelvic floor muscles. That's a goal well worth striving for.

Exercise can help with erectile dysfunction in a number of ways. As well as helping you to lose weight and generally feel better about yourself, exercise improves blood flow all over the body, and particularly to the penis. It's also a great mood lifter, and can counteract any stress or depression you may be experiencing as a result of your condition. And if you perform specific pelvic floor exercises, as well as exercising generally, you'll increase your chances of enjoying a normal sex life once more.

Perhaps the best benefit of exercise is that, unlike Viagra, or other drugs which may be used to treat erectile dysfunction, it doesn't have any side effects, other than helping you to lose weight and feel fitter and healthier than ever before. If you don't exercise enough, maybe you should make an effort to be more active, for the sake of both your health and your sex life.

Regular cardio vascular exercises

Aside from increasing energy levels, improving muscle tone and reducing blood pressure, performing cardio vascular exercises on a regular basis can help reduce the risk for erectile dysfunction or if a man is already suffering from it, address it. Aside from allowing a man to achieve and maintain a healthy weight (remember obesity and its relationship to erectile dysfunction?), doing so can help a man get enough sleep, manage stress well, feel better about himself and improve heart health – all of which can help address erectile dysfunction issues. Such exercises include:

-Brisk walking;

-Dancing;

-Exercising on an elliptical trainer;

-Rowing;

-Running;

-Swimming; and

-Tae Bo.

To maximize the health benefits of regular cardio vascular exercising, the ideal duration and frequency is 20 to 30 minutes and 4 to 5 times per week, respectively. As mentioned in an earlier chapter, don't overdo it nor take it too easy. If it's your first time to do cardio, consult with a doctor first to assess the optimal duration, intensity and frequency for you.

Lifting weights

One of the best ways to improve blood flow to the penis is to improving the health of blood vessels' inner lining called the endothelium. A healthy endothelium, according to prominent urology professor Dr. Wane Hellstrom, M.D., of the Tulane University School of Medicine, helps in improving a man's erections. Weight lifting or resistance training exercises can also help improve a man's endothelium health and consequently, blood flow to the penis.

In more ways than one, weight lifting can also help address psychological erectile dysfunction. How? Lifting weights makes a man physically stronger and look better (more muscular) ala Ryan Gosling or Ryan Reynolds. Looking better and being stronger can significantly improve a man's self-confidence and the way he sees himself as a sex object, both of which can stoke the fire of sexiness within and improve his ability to feel sexually aroused. And when a man is sexually aroused, you know what happens next.

Yoga

Erectile dysfunction, especially psychological ones, are brought about by excess stress and fatigue. One of the best ways to manage and control both is by fostering a very strong connection between body and mind, which can be done through exercises like yoga.

Yoga has been shown in many studies to be effective in terms of reducing stress and general tension of the body as well as in terms of improving one's breathing. It's also generally helpful in improving a person's feeling of being well, which is also important for sexual arousal.

Yoga doesn't just help address psychological erectile dysfunction – it also helps address physiological ones. It's because some forms of yoga exercises can help improve the pelvic region's blood circulation. Since erections are primarily about blood flow in that region, it can help men's penises to "stand up and pay attention."

Salsa

Let's face it, many people would like to have their cakes and eat them too by combining exercise and fun all in one session. It's also worth noting that not everyone finds lifting weights and doing cardio to be fun. The answer? Try something like dancing – particularly salsa!

The beautiful thing about salsa dancing apart from being a good cardiovascular exercise is that it's something that a couple can enjoy together. Not only does it burn much calories, it can also be so much fun with the music and the opportunity to develop more intimacy between both partners, which can translate to a much better sexual relationship. Improved blood flow and emotional well-being – what more can you ask for in an exercise, eh?

Chapter 11

How Diet Can Help With Erectile Dysfunction

'You are what you eat.' It's an old saying, and like many old sayings, there's a lot of truth in it. How does eating apply to erectile dysfunction? Well, in two ways really. Often, potency problems may have an underlying medical or nutritional contributory factor. Your lack of erection may be a sign of other problems, rather than just something on its own, so you need to look at your whole lifestyle and find out if you can improve things at that end. And of course, some foods are actually known to have aphrodisiac properties, so it's worth including those in your diet. If you think diet is just something that women have to concern themselves with, think again. If your eyes glaze over at the thought of nutrition and other boring stuff like that, it may help to think of your in the same way you think of your car. After all, your body is an amazing machine too, and it deserves your love and devotion just as much as your car – even more so, actually, because your car doesn't have to last you a lifetime, but your body does, so it needs to be treated with respect to get the best performance out of it in all departments. See where this is going? When you refuel your car, you use the most appropriate fuel to keep it in good running order. You wouldn't put rubbish in your car, so if you're already putting rubbish in your body in the form of processed foods and foods high in fats, sugars and salts, maybe it's time to take a detailed look at your diet and make the changes that can help to get your body working better and your sex life back on track.

First and foremost, a healthy diet reduces the risk of many factors which can impact on erectile dysfunction. This is because one of the physical reasons for the condition is vascular problems which restrict the flow of blood to the penis. This blood flow is important in achieving an erection and sustaining it through lovemaking, so it's important to address your diet and see if it is heart healthy, because basically a diet that is good for the heart is also good for the penis!

Factors that can impact on heart health, such as being overweight, having high blood pressure, high cholesterol or high levels of blood triglycerides can all contribute to vascular problems. One way to instantly improve this situation is to cut down on the processed foods in your diet, or better yet, try to cut them out altogether. Make a pledge to eat only recognizable food, and you will more or less guarantee to be pretty much eliminating processed and junk foods from your diet.

Recent research suggests that in 80% of erectile dysfunction cases, the problem is vascular. Not only does this create problems in the bedroom, it could be an indication and a warning sign of a more serious condition such as heart disease. Following the right diet can help minimize the risk factors for heart disease, and at the same time, it can help with your potency problems.

The Mediterranean Diet

Many doctors and dieticians recommend the Mediterranean Diet as one of the healthiest in the world. More a healthy eating plan than a diet as such, it's high in the antioxidants that help to prevent heart disease and other chronic conditions. Recent research in Athens, Greece has concluded that men who follow the Mediterranean Diet are likely to have healthier vascular systems and fewer problems with erectile dysfunction. Remember this is not a problem that is the exclusive preserve of older men – young men have the problem too, and in the majority of cases, it's down to vascular health.

The Mediterranean Diet consists of fresh, in season foods, with the emphasis on fish and low fat proteins such as poultry and eggs. Olive oil is at the heart of it, and it's one of the healthiest oils there is. Following the Mediterranean Diet will boost your metabolism and help you to lose any excess pounds you may be carrying, as well as lowering your blood pressure and regulating blood glucose levels. All of this is great news for your vascular system.

The Mediterranean Diet involves eating natural foods such as whole grains, fruits, vegetables, limited red meat, plenty of heart healthy oily fish and some dairy products such as yogurt and cheese. Healthy fats come from nuts and olive oil in moderation. You can also enjoy a little wine. One aspect of the diet is that it's good for kidney health, and that may also help to solve the problem of erectile dysfunction, since as well as vascular issues, men may also have problems with urination which may be contributing to the condition.

Because it's high in fruit and vegetable consumption, the Mediterranean Diet is also high in antioxidants. That's the nutrients that mop up the free radicals in the system which can cause cancer, heart disease and other chronic conditions. Studies suggest that around on third of men with erectile dysfunction can get back to fully functioning within two years, simply by following the Mediterranean Diet and incorporating more exercise into their lives.

A number of factors contribute to this success. Perhaps the main thing is that a healthy diet can help men lose excess weight. Too much belly fat is known to lower testosterone levels, which can contribute to loss of sexual function. Also, many fresh foods have anti-inflammatory properties, and people who are overweight often suffer from internal inflammation, which can impact on general health as well as sexual performance.

Foods that can help overcome erectile dysfunction

As well as following a healthy diet like the Mediterranean Diet, there are certain foods that can help overcome erectile dysfunction due to their specific nutrients. Eating healthily can take care of your general health, including your vascular health, which is an important component of addressing your potency problems, so that's a great start. Now let's look at some of the foods that can help, and why they are so important in your diet. These are not necessarily aphrodisiac foods, but they do contain vitamins and nutrients that can improve your sexual health, so put them on your shopping list, if you don't already have them in the house.

Beans, seeds, legumes and other proteins

Protein is a very necessary nutrient. It's needed for just about every bodily function, including cell repair and renewal, and it helps build muscle and keep you feeling fuller for longer, which is great when you're trying to lose excess weight. The thing with proteins, whether it comes from animal or plant sources, is that it contains amino acids which may not be essential for health, but can certainly bring about improvements in your physical condition.

Arginine is one of these amino acids. It's essential for children, but not necessarily for adults. However, one important function of arginine is that it helps to increase blood flow by dilating the blood vessels. As has already been mentioned, that's important for vascular health and normal sexual function in males. How does that work? Simply put, arginine helps the body to produce nitric oxide, which is instrumental in relaxing the blood vessels, making for more efficient circulation and better overall health, as well as improving sexual function.

So if you can include plenty of arginine containing foods in your diet, you can help yourself to a more satisfying sex life. Foods that are high in arginine are mostly protein-based, so eat more beans, legumes and seeds, lean meat and poultry, dairy products and oily fish. Top arginine containing foods are tuna, salmon, trout, sesame seeds and walnuts. It's in green peppers too, as well as quinoa, oats and wheat or rice based cereals.

It may be a little difficult to ensure you're getting enough arginine, since it's not something that's listed on the nutrient panels of various foods. However, if you aim for a minimum of 56 grams of protein each day, you should be getting enough arginine to promote vascular health and dilate those blood vessels.

Fruits and Vegetables

If you've ever been tempted to buy drugs online to address your erectile dysfunction issues, or if you've thought about asking your doctor to prescribe them, you should know something. Most of the drugs for this condition are based on the action of nitrates in the body, and their ability to relax the blood vessels, allowing for better blood flow into the penis.

The good news is, unless you have a problem with nitrate absorption, you can get all you need from eating the right kinds of vegetables. Leafy green vegetables such as spinach and celery are high in nitrates, and so is watermelon.

Lycopene is also good for relaxing those pesky blood vessels, and you can get that from tomatoes and pink grapefruit, among other things. A word of caution though – if you're taking statins for high cholesterol, or anti coagulants such as warfarin, steer clear of grapefruit. For everyone else, lycopene works best when combined with oily foods, so why not make up a salad with tuna, avocado and tomatoes, and fight erectile dysfunction in a tasty, healthy, and above all natural way?

Cranberries are good to go for enhanced sexual health as well. They can help clear up any urinary tract infections or inflammation which may be exacerbating your performance problems.

Shellfish

Oysters have been talked up as an aphrodisiac since time immemorial. And the reason why is that they're high in zinc. Zinc is necessary for producing testosterone, and if your levels are low, that could be contributing to your potency problems. The truth is, oysters and other shellfish can bring on that loving feeling in both men and women, so go ahead and tuck in.

Not keen on oysters? They are probably the best source of zinc – just one oyster can provide the recommended daily allowance. Don't fret if you don't like them though – other seafood such as crab, clams, lobsters and mussels are also good sources of zinc. Organize a seafood treat at least once a week. On the days you don't go in for seafood, meat, nuts and seeds and fortified cereals can help keep your zinc levels topped up to testosterone producing levels. And of course, they're all foods you'll be eating anyway if you're following the Mediterranean Diet.

Dark chocolate

Lots of recent studies have come up with good reasons to eat dark chocolate – especially high quality dark chocolate. It seems that this former guilty pleasure can also help with erectile dysfunction, due to its high flavonoid content. Flavonoids are the substances that repair cell damage in plants, and they're pretty good for humans too, since they can help lower blood pressure and cholesterol, both of which can have an adverse impact on sexual health as well as general health. Of course, you need to remember that even though it's good for you, chocolate is still high in calories and fat, so don't be too indulgent.

While no particular food can prevent or treat erectile dysfunction, it's clear from nutritional knowledge and recent studies that a healthy diet can work wonders in improving general health and vascular health in particular. Remember around 80% of erectile dysfunction cases have nothing to do with age, strength, sexual prowess or anything else. The root cause is problems in the blood vessels that supply the penis. Following a heart healthy diet like the Mediterranean Diet can go a long way towards addressing those problems, and set you on the way to improved sexual health, particularly when a healthy diet is combined with regular exercise.

Foods that are high in nitrates can be as effective in treating erectile dysfunction as many of the drugs prescribed for the condition, since their main function is to improve circulation to allow unrestricted blood flow into the penis to achieve and maintain an erection. Wouldn't you rather eat yourself back to sexual health than pop pills which may have unwanted and unpleasant side effects? Take a long look at your diet, and make the necessary changes, and you'll soon get your mojo back.

Bradley Martin

Chapter 12
Supplementation

Since a big chunk of erectile dysfunction is physiological, it stands to follow that good nutrition is key to addressing the issue. Great nutrition is all about wise eating habits and choices. Unfortunately, it isn't always possible to get all the necessary nutrients by simply eating the right foods. Often times, supplementation is needed. Eating right for addressing or reducing the risks for erectile dysfunction may require taking supplements for optimal penile health. Truth is, natural supplements, e.g., herbs, have been used since time immemorial in addressing erectile issues by African and Chinese cultures.

Compared to prescription medications for treating erectile dysfunctions such as Cialis (tadalafil), Levitra (vardenafil) and Viagra (sildenafil), supplements don't have as extensive studies or tests to back up their efficacy claims. As the amount and type of active ingredients among different erectile dysfunction supplements may vary, their side effects do so as well.

Because supplementation can be quite helpful to address erectile dysfunctions, here's a guide for choosing erectile dysfunction supplements:

Generally safe, with positive results from studies of people

> ➢ DHEA: There's some amount of evidence showing its ability to address erectile dysfunction. Generally safe at low doses but have been reported to cause acne in some cases.

> ➢ L-ARGININE: There's some evidence establishing its ability to stimulate wider blood vessel opening to increase blood flow. In some cases, it's been reported to cause diarrhea, cramps and nausea. Avoid taking together with Viagra.

> ➢ GINSENG: Panax ginseng has been shown in one study to improve sexual function for men who suffer from erectile dysfunction. It's cream form – applied topically – can help prevent premature ejaculation. Although generally safe for short-term use, using panax ginseng as a supplement can cause insomnia for some people.

With positive results from studies of people but higher risk

➤ YOHIMBE: Some clinical studies have shown yohimbe to help improve erectile dysfunctions brought about by anti-depressant medications but have also been reported to cause relatively serious side effects in some people like anxiety, irregular heartbeat and elevated blood pressure. As such, this supplement should only be taken with approval from a licensed physician.

No significant studies on people

➤ GINGKO: This herbal supplement has good potential to improve penile blood flow but no solid evidence exists regarding claims of effectively addressing erectile dysfunction. A potential side effect of this herbal supplement is risk for bleeding.

➤ HORNY GOAT WEED (EPIMEDIUM): Although the leaves of this herb contain ingredients that are used for better sexual performance, there are no established studies on people that support the belief in its efficacy. A bonus side effect of this herbal supplement is it can help lower blood pressure.

Other non-prescription herbal alternatives

Several herbal products that claim to be the "natural" Viagra proliferate the market. The thing is, these products have undisclosed quantities of potent ingredients that are also found in their supposed synthetic counterparts and thus have higher risks for unwanted side effects. In fact, some of these products actually contain the very drugs that their supposed synthetic counterparts have that require a doctor's prescription to consume! In this case, it's best to be very vigilant in taking "herbal" erectile dysfunction supplements from manufacturers that aren't well known or don't have a good reputation in the market. Even if the FDA has banned such "herbal" supplements, they continue to proliferate illegally.

Remember, it's not enough that manufacturers claim that theirs are herbal – it's easy to claim such stuff without backing them up. Because it's practically impossible for ordinary consumers like you and I to distinguish, it's best to stick with relatively more expensive brands of herbal supplements from well-established manufacturers.

Being labeled "herbal" doesn't necessarily mean safe. Remember, they may be say taken as is but some of them may react negatively if taken with other medications. As such, it's best to consult with a licensed physician first prior to taking such supplements for erectile dysfunction, especially when taking regular medications.

Online purchase risks

With the proliferation of many online stores these days and the convenience shopping on such stores brings, no wonder many people choose to buy their supplements online. Beware though – many supplements for erectile dysfunction that are sold online these days contain ingredients that need prescription or worse, are undisclosed.

Many men who purchase erectile dysfunction supplements online think these are safe because of the nice packaging. These are often labeled as "all-natural" or "safer than prescription medicines but are just as effective." The scary truth is often times, the label tells a different story than the content. The worse thing that can happen is that these supplements contain dangerous ingredients that aren't on the label. In fact, the United States Food And Drugs Administration (FDA) – through its Internet and Health Fraud division – conducted an online survey that revealed more than 1/3 of erectile dysfunction supplements purchased online contained prescription grade ingredients and other similar substances that weren't even disclosed.

Two of these are the ingredients sildenafil and vardenafil (or substances very similar to these), the active ingredients for Viagra and Levitra, respectively. If people who have issues with Viagra and Levitra take these supplements thinking they're safer than the two prescription medicines, they may be in for a rude awakening as they suffer from side effects that they're trying to avoid in the first place.

What's more, even if the men taking these supplements have no issues with Viagra or Levitra, it's possible for them to suffer adverse side effects if they're taking medicines that don't mix well with the 2 prescription medicines' active ingredients that aren't disclosed in the supplements. For example, if a person is taking prescription medicine that contains nitrates, taking supplements that unknowingly contain sildenafil (an active component of Viagra) may bring down his blood pressure dangerously low. Nitrates are a common ingredient in prescription medicines used to treat or manage heart disease, high cholesterol, high blood pressure and diabetes and incidentally, men who are being treated for these conditions also suffer from erectile dysfunction.

Here's a list of supplements sold in the market that purportedly treat erectile dysfunction and improve sexual performance. This is by no means an extensive list.

➤ 4EVERON

- Actra-Rx
- Actra-Sx
- Adam Free
- Blue Steel
- Energy Max
- Erextra
- Hero
- HS Joy of Love
- Lady Shangai
- Libidus
- Liviro3
- Lycium Barbarum L.
- Nasutra
- Naturalë Super Plus
- NaturalUp
- Neophase
- Rhino V Max
- Shangai Regular, also marketed as Shangai Chaojimengnan
- Shangai Ultra
- Shangai Ultra X
- Strong Testis
- Super Shangai
- True Man

➤ V.Max

➤ Vigor-25

➤ Xiadafil VIP tablets (Lots 6K029 and 6K209-SEI only)

➤ Yilishen

➤ Zimaxx

Non-oral solutions for erectile dysfunction

Until recently, medical or supplemental treatments for erectile dysfunction were taken orally. Although those may work well for many, there are some men who aren't predisposed to the ingredients of such medicines or supplements, especially those who take prescription medicines that contain nitrates. Oral treatments may also have side effects that can negate the erection benefits offered.

Now, non-oral treatments are available for erectile dysfunctions as an alternative to oral treatments. They vary in efficacy and side effects. To help you sift through them, here's a list of the most popular topical solutions for erectile dysfunction:

➤ AndroGel: Many cases of erectile dysfunctions are caused by low testosterone levels. One of the most popular ways of addressing this deficiency is testosterone replacement but technically, it doesn't help men with normal levels of testosterone and those who suffer from erectile dysfunction. Testosterone can also be delivered by skin application via AndroGel – testosterone in a gel. Some of the potential side effects worth noting are emotional instability, acne and headache.

➤ Alprostadil: This kind of topical solution is classified as a vasodilator, substances that can help blood vessels to expand and improve blood flow. Since erectile dysfunction is physically a blood flow issue, Alprostadil is used for treating erectile dysfunction and is administered directly via injection into the penis or suppository insertion into the urethra. In has a reported efficacy rate of about 80%. There are no known side effects.

Alprostadil is also available as a topically applied solution, which spares men from penile scarring, bleeding and bruising. Tests have confirmed that it helps in most erectile dysfunction cases with minimal and tolerable side effects.

Chapter 13

Is Lack of Confidence Causing Erectile Dysfunction?

So far, this book has examined various physical causes of erectile dysfunction, and discussed some of the treatment options, including diet and lifestyle changes. But sometimes, there may not be a physical cause for the problem. If you're in your 30s, fit and well, with great vascular function and you're not carrying any extra weight or suffering from a chronic condition, yet you still have problems achieving and maintaining an erection, maybe you need to look beyond the physical.

Sometimes, lack of confidence can be the problem. It doesn't necessarily have to be sexually related either. It may stem from a fear of not being good enough for someone you care deeply about. You want to please them so much – not just sexually, but in every way possible. You want to be a friend, lover and provider. They are the most important person in your life, and you want to be the most important person in theirs. The problem is, you want it so badly, that you doubt your ability to deliver.

You may have a great job that pays well, that you enjoy, and you're good at, as well as being highly regarded by your boss and colleagues. You may even have a lovely home, and no money worries. You're a good looking guy, not carrying too much weight, and you've still got all your own teeth. And you have the right work/life balance, so what's stopping you from enjoying a great relationship with the woman you love? Frankly, you are! You're trying to be the perfect partner in every way, and there is no such animal. Nobody is perfect. All anyone can do, whatever their advantages or disadvantages, is to do their best. The problem is, you may feel that your best just isn't good enough, and that's when the problems start.

It may not even start with sexual performance – chances are that everything in the bedroom is rosy at first. It's as you get to know each other better and move towards commitment that confidence issues may arise. The thing is, when a relationship gets to this stage, you start to think about the future. Until now, you've been enjoying each other's company – and hopefully each other's bodies – and all the thinking you've done is about how much you enjoy being together and how you can't wait for the next time.

Once you start thinking about making a life together, anxieties and doubts start to creep in. Not about your partner – you're as sure as you can be that she's the one. Your doubts revolve around yourself, and your ability to be the partner she wants and deserves.

The way to get over this is to focus your thoughts on something else, other than yourself and your perceived failings. It can be a person or a thing, as long as it stops you thinking about yourself and therefore undermining your confidence even further. Some psychologists recommend losing yourself in a logic puzzle, or a difficult cryptic crossword or Sudoku. If you're not into puzzles, try burying yourself in a really good book, or even a video game. The important thing is that every time you feel your thoughts turning inwardly, you distract them before you get into that vicious cycle of doubt and anxiety, where you convince yourself that you're a failure, and it eventually becomes a self-fulfilling prophecy.

If you can get involved in something that holds your attention, you can break the cycle of negative thoughts and feelings. It may not feel like it, but you can actually control your thoughts and feelings, and take them in another direction. While it's all too easy to slide into a spiral of negative thinking that can result in erectile dysfunction, it's more difficult to train yourself to think positively, and turn your attitude around. Difficult – but by no means impossible.

The problem is, even if negativity doesn't start in the bedroom, that's where it's likely to end up, unless you can break the cycle. Men – unlike women – are not good about talking about their problems, especially when it comes to sex, because so much is invested in sexual performance, as far as most men are concerned. If there are problems in the bedroom, they see themselves as failures – no matter how successful they are in other areas of their lives, men who can't satisfy themselves and their partners sexually consider themselves to be failures. When it comes down to it, the good job, the nice house, the fancy car and the money in the bank count for nothing if they can't get an erection.

There are only two requirements for an erection – you need to be aroused, and you also need to be relaxed. If you are lacking in confidence, for whatever reason, you are not likely to be relaxed, and if your self-confidence issues have been ongoing for some time, you probably can't get aroused either.

Things you can do to increase self-confidence

Many people don't realize it but self-confidence is like physical muscles – it can be developed through training. It can get better with continuous use or get weak as it's left unused. The following are good ways to exercise your self-confidence muscles and develop them even more:

➤ Continue learning new things. One of the ways you can feel confident is by knowing things that most other people don't, including sexual tips and tricks. Who says learning can't be fun, eh?

➤ Step out of yourself and be a better person by doing something good for other people. How does this help develop self-confidence? By regularly thinking and doing something good for other people, you train yourself to be selfless and the less self-centered you become, the less conscious you become about your perceived "shortcomings", which lessens your tendency to be down on yourself.

➤ Hit the weights at the gym. If you want to look as buffed and macho as Hugh Jackman, Ryan Gosling and Ryan Reynolds, skip the marathons and hit the weights. You don't build muscles with cardio – you do it with resistance training. I know it sounds superficial but hey, looking buffed and macho can do a lot to boost self-confidence.

➤ Get out there and meet people even if you're an introvert. One of the best ways to overcome fear is by facing them head on and for most men who lack self-confidence, one of their greatest fears is reaching out and meeting new people. Confident people aren't afraid to make new friends and making new friends does wonders to boost self-confidence. So next time you're at a social event, get out of your comfort zone and meet new people.

➤ Know what matters most to you. There are times that not knowing what you value most can lead to low self-esteem. How? By being all over the place, you may spread yourself too thin to achieve anything significant. By knowing what matters most to you, you can focus your time, effort and resources on those priorities and increase your chances of achieving meaningful things, which can do wonders for self-confidence.

➤ Identify things that are harmful to you and your self-esteem that aren't really needed in your life and make an effort to get rid of them. Are you in an emotionally draining relationship with a girlfriend? Break up with her and find your joy elsewhere. Life's too short to be too preoccupied with unnecessary emotional stress and self-esteem bubble bursters.

➤ Do something you absolutely fear. Just keep it to safe and healthy ones, ok? Overcoming serious fears help bump up self-confidences several notches. For example, people who have had near-death experiences tend to become more sociable and confident knowing that they cheated something that most other people fear most – death. Try eating an exotic dish that most people absolutely fear eating, go bungee jumping or approach that hot chick sitting at the bar to introduce yourself and get her digits.

➤ Do some self-searching to identify thought patterns or habits that normally cause you to feel unconfident about yourself. After you've done so, imagine that someone close to you is thinking the same way and as a result, experience low self esteem. How would you talk them out of feeling that way? Do the same to yourself.

➤ Identify the things that really make you intellectually and emotionally come alive and make time to regularly indulge in them. Often times, doing the things that make you alive translate directly to higher self-esteem.

➤ Step out of the roles you play in life that you're squeezing into just to please other people but aren't really cut out for. If for example, you're trying to be an insurance salesman because your parents expect you to become one just like your dad but being one isn't really your thing, there's nothing wrong in dropping it in favor of something you really want to do and know are more equipped to succeed in. Continuously trying to conform to others' expectations of you at the expense of what you really want (assuming what you want isn't sinful or illegal) is a sure fire way to emasculate yourself and is the figurative equivalent of being neutered.

➤ Develop the skill of catching yourself every time you say or think that you're not good enough, talented enough or endowed enough to succeed. Learn to replace those self-depreciating scripts with confidence building ones. One way to help you do this is by regularly basking in the memories of past successes. As long as you don't overdo it, you remind yourself that you are worth something and that you are capable of achieving things, which can significantly help you have a healthy self-confidence.

➤ Stop the habit of making important decisions without deliberately thinking through them. By thinking through such decisions and being deliberate with them, you reduce your risk of making wrong ones and consequently, increase your chances of making good and successful ones. Thinking through includes acknowledging your concerns and doubts in order to have as much of your decision bases covered. There's a differences between being pessimistic and being pragmatic. Be the latter, not the former

➤ Stop beating yourself up over past mistakes such as wrong decisions, inability to perform as expected or passing up on a great opportunity because doing so won't make things better but will only make them worse. The best thing to do is learn from them and realize that everybody makes mistakes every now and then. When similar situations crop up, you'll be more confident knowing what caused you to screw up a similar situation in the past and that you're now in a position to avoid making the same mistake.

➤ Don't confuse being scared with not being confident. Even the most confident people can still be scared at times. I know of a person who preaches to crowds of thousands every week and still feel so nervous before going up on stage that sometimes he pukes before going to the auditorium. It's ok to be scared – it's an acknowledgment that you're not perfect. What's not ok is not to be confident.

➤ There will always be people who'll make you feel unsure of yourself with the things they say to and about you. There's a difference between constructive feedback and outright putting you down and you don't have to put up with the latter. Either tell them to stop putting you down or leave them. You'll be much better without them anyway.

➤ This may sound unrelated but trust me it is – flirt! Why? The better you get at it with women, the more confident you'll feel about yourself. Trust me.

➢ Be vulnerable to others. Being vulnerable allows you to overcome one of the biggest fears for most people – rejection. As you master the art of vulnerability, you don't just master the fear of rejection, you'll find that people will draw closer to you and be vulnerable too. You have the side benefit of enjoying more intimate relationships on top of increased self-confidence.

➢ Be humble and admit it when you're wrong. Confidence for the sake of confidence is a fake one and won't last long. It's like building a mansion on sand. What you'd want is a self-confidence that sticks and lasts. Admitting your mistake has the same effect as being vulnerable – you let go of your fear of rejection and as a bonus, you earn other people's respect and confidence too.

➢ Regularly see yourself in your mind's eye (visualize) as the successful and confident person you want to be. Truth is, our subconscious minds are the ones responsible for our regular behavior and feelings and it can't distinguish what's real or not. By visualizing your successful self often, you feed the idea of a successful you to your subconscious mind and over time, it will act out that confident self you've fed it.

➢ Learn to ask for help. Why? You wont' be able to do everything by yourself. By enlisting the help of others, you'll be able to achieve more meaningful goals, which directly increase your self-confidence. Knowing you have other people to back you up in important tasks can also make you feel more confident about taking bigger responsibilities.

➤ Take risks. No meaningful achievements were ever accomplished without taking risks and the higher the risk, the bigger the potential success. If you want to be a successful person and feel more confident, you'll definitely have to be comfortable taking risks. Just take well-calculated ones though. Taking risks doesn't necessarily mean gambling your life and safety away.

➤ Spend more time with people who make you feel appreciated, important and significant. You can only go so far convincing yourself of such and the validation of others is a very powerful tool for building and increasing self-confidence.

➤ Fake it till you make it. As you learned earlier in the CBE (cognitive behavior emotion) model, actions can go a long way towards influencing your thoughts and emotions. If you want to feel and think confident, start acting the part.

➤ Stop comparing yourself to others. It's a well-known fact that there will always be someone who'll be better at you at what you do best. As such, know that it's very counterproductive to compare yourself to other people, regardless if the people you're comparing yourself to are "superior" or "inferior" to you. The only person you should compare yourself to is yourself.

➤ Speak your mind during group discussions more often. For many people, speaking in front of many others can be quite a scary experience. If you deliberately go against your fear of speaking in public by speaking out your mind every time you're in a group, especially a large one such as a seminar or class, you weaken the fear and will start to experience a sense of self-confidence you've never experienced before. Face the fear to kill it and be more confident!

➤ Learn to value yourself for who you are and not who people want you to be. Live your life according to your values and beliefs and start experiencing unparalleled freedom from people's expectations, which will make you a truly confident person.

What confident people don't do

For many people, confidence is equal to being proud or self-centered. Nothing can be farther from the truth. The fact is, people who are truly confident about themselves don't go around bragging about themselves or tooting their own horns. If any, confident people are either thought of initially as shy or indifferent. Shy because they're often silent about their accomplishments knowing they don't have anything to prove. Indifferent because confident people couldn't care less about what goes on around them or about what others think of them.

To help you become more confident, here's a list of some of the things truly confident people don't do:

➤ They avoid humiliating or judging others because not only is it wrong, they are secure enough with who they are that they don't feel the need to put others down just bring themselves up. In fact, they do the opposite: they lift other people up because they're not insecure.

➤ They don't try to bring attention to themselves because again, they're secure with who they are that they don't feel the need to be noticed.

➤ They also don't try to dismiss any attention that's given to them freely. Because of the same sense of security, they're able to graciously and comfortably receive attention from others.

➤ They don't brag about themselves or whatever they've achieved. Why? Why not? They don't need others' approval to feel good about themselves so they don't feel the need to brag.

➤ They don't dismiss others' compliments about them and their achievements either. In fact, being confident in who they are allows them to comfortably receive and acknowledge other peoples' praises without letting those get into their heads.

➤ They're not critical. Because they're secure, they don't feel the need to criticize others and as such, they ooze positivity and charisma, which attracts more people to them and make them feel even more confident.

➤ They don't just talk about themselves. An offshoot of being confident about one's identity and person is the ability to talk more about others than one's self. They are genuinely interested in others and it shows in them asking much about others and genuinely wanting to know others better and praise them. As such, confident people make for great conversationalists.

➤ They don't fuss over the small things. Because confident people are secure with themselves, they're also confident about being able to handle situations and thus don't make a fuss when things go wrong. Such confidence leads to a calmness in the face of challenges, whether big or small, which inspires the people around them to be as calm and collected.

➤ Confident people don't focus on things that aren't important. A big chunk of being confident is knowing what are the truly important things to focus on and as such, they're able to stick to what's really important and maximize their time, effort and resources.

➤ They don't break promises and commitments. Confident people know when to commit and promise and when not to because they know the things that they're truly capable of accomplishing. As such, confident people rarely overpromise and under deliver but usually under promise and over deliver. By doing the latter, they minimize the risk of broken promises and commitments.

Bradley Martin

Chapter 14

Other Therapies for Erectile Dysfunction

Massage

In other countries, you may have heard or read of stories about a massage therapy that's used to enhance men's sexual performance. That's true – there is such a massage, especially in Asia. It's called prostate massage therapy. In centuries past, many Asian wives employed the services of monks or doctors to give their husbands prostate massages to ensure optimal sexual performance.

These days, prostate massage therapy is looked at as more than just sexual performance enhancing treatment. It's also considered as a vital practice for enhancing and maintaining prostate health. Prostate massage therapy is also used these days as a means for relief of symptoms of prostatitis and enlarged prostate glands and as a way of maintaining good sexual and prostate health. Still, it's best to consult with a medical professional before deciding to undergo this kind of therapy to determine if it's safe for you.

Just how are prostate massages done? It's done by massaging the prostate internally or externally in several ways. Internally, a lubricated and gloved finger is inserted inside the man's anus and is pressed against his prostate gland. Either a doctor, himself or his partner can do this. The person administering this massage then carefully probes for the prostate gland, which will feel like a tiny ball. The massage is done by applying light pressure and releasing said pressure on different areas of the prostate. Prostatic fluid is released at the end of the man's penis when pressure is applied at the center of the gland.

An alternative to using a lubricated gloved finger is an internal prostate massager. This kind of massager has a lubricated part, which is inserted in the anus to massage the prostate.

Externally, a prostate massage is done by applying gentle pressure to the perineum – the area between a man's scrotum and anus – using a finger. This pressure is applied along the entire length between the anus and scrotum for optimal massage benefits. An external prostate massaging instrument can also be used to do the same.

This therapy is also called prostate milking because doing so helps release prostatic fluid out of the penis, which helps reduce prostate inflammation by opening up channels in the gland. This type of massage helps improve erectile performance by improving the pelvis' muscle tone.

One advantage of doing this massage is that it can be administered in the comfort of one's home. Still, a doctor's clearance is best prior to having this done.

Speaking of prostate massage devices, it's important that one is able to get the real deal and not just repackaged dildos or other sex toys made to look like prostate massagers. One way to do so is to pay close attention to the packaging, particularly who the manufacturer or marketer is, prior to getting one.

Internal prostate massagers, i.e. inserted inside the anus, may or may not have vibrating functions. Because the prostate can be rather fragile, you don't want to get an unsafe prostate massager that vibrates like a jackhammer, right? Right!

A good prostate massager is the Sonic Prostate Massager that features a sonic wave massage function for stimulating the prostate area, relax it, bring down inflammation and enhance fluids and blood flow in the pelvic area, which can help treat erectile dysfunction. Other internal prostate massagers utilize non-sonic waves, i.e. vibration, to massage and stimulate the prostate.

Eternal prostate massagers are, as the name says, not inserted inside the anus. Men can use this by sitting down. They're made to massage a particular spot called the perineum.

Using such a device can certainly make it easier to massage the prostate for treating erectile dysfunction. Look for prostate massagers that offer money-back guarantees as this is a sign of a quality device. Only a manufacturer who is supremely confident about their product's quality will be sane enough to offer such a guarantee. And when you start using it for erectile dysfunction, be patient. It takes at least a few weeks for the benefits of daily prostate massaging to become obvious.

Counseling

Men, unlike women, find it difficult to talk through their problems. Often, they have difficulty even admitting they have a problem in the first place, let alone talking about it to someone they care about. This is when it may be handy to talk to someone who is not close to you but has experience in counseling people with sexual problems. Even if there is a physical cause for erectile dysfunction, it can often sap a man's sexual confidence. Maybe an unfortunate sexual encounter or encounters in the past is responsible for the lack of confidence that is causing problems in the here and now.

The thing with confidence is that it's so easy to lose and yet so difficult to regain. Sometimes it never returns. Talking with someone who is non-judgmental, practical and a good listener may help you overcome your lack of confidence and start feeling good about yourself again. Sometimes just saying stuff out loud takes away its ability to cause you worry, emotional pain and difficulty. Nothing is ever as bad as it seems once it is out in the open and being talked about.

Acknowledging the problem goes a long way towards finding the solution, and counselors are skilled in the art of drawing out your true feelings and helping you to examine and analyze them. If your self-help methods of rebuilding your confidence aren't succeeding, maybe you need to seek the help of a counselor. It should be someone you can engage with and feel comfortable with, due to the highly personal subject matter.

Your doctor may be able to recommend someone suitable, or if you don't feel you can discuss such intimate things with a complete stranger, there are a number of online counseling services available. Whatever type of counselor you decide to use, check out their credentials and ask to see testimonials, so you can set your mind at rest that they are qualified to help you, and have helped others with similar problems in the past.

Hypnotherapy

These days, people are trying hypnosis for all sorts of lifestyle problems – quitting smoking, losing weight, getting over bereavement, fear of flying and sexual problems, among many others. Before taking this route, you need to be positive that this is what you want to do, and you also need to have confidence in the ability of the hypnotherapist. In other words, you need an open mind and trust in your practitioner, because if you don't believe hypnosis will do any good, you're setting yourself up for failure before you even try.

Hypnosis has proved successful for many people where other methods have failed, so it's worth a try. The hypnotherapist can address all the mental problems that are causing your erectile dysfunction, including lack of confidence and anxiety, depression and low self-esteem. It is likely that you will need several sessions before any improvement is noticed, so be prepared for that, and don't expect a quick fix.

The hypnotherapist may use one or more techniques to help you, or a combination of several methods. Some may involve suggestion and instructions, while others may be aimed at resolving the underlying cause or causes of the problem. Make sure your chosen therapist discusses all available options, and the reasons why they may or may not work in your case.

Sometimes the treatment may involve delving into your subconscious mind – particularly if there is no physical cause for your problem, and you can't figure out a solid psychological or emotional cause. You need to realize that you may find yourself having to confront things that have been buried – possibly for many years – and you need to be ready to deal with what you may discover about yourself and other people during your treatment. Any or all of the above tactics may be able to help you restore your confidence, to a point where you can contemplate sexual intercourse without wondering whether you will manage to get and maintain an erection. If you don't feel confident enough to help yourself, don't be afraid or ashamed to call in the experts. Everyone needs help from someone at some stage in their life, and you are no different. Better to go for counseling or therapy than live with erectile dysfunction for longer than you need to.

Bradley Martin

Chapter 15

Could A Sex Therapist Help With Erectile Dysfunction?

Sex therapists seem to be everywhere these days – on chat shows, online, on the radio, and even in your high street. You may be living next door to a sex therapist and not even know it! So, what is a sex therapist, what do they do, and can they help with erectile dysfunction? Here are some of the answers to your questions. Only you can decide if a sex therapist is appropriate in your particular case, and this chapter should help you to make that decision.

What is a sex therapist?

A properly qualified sex therapist – and that's the only type you should consider using - is likely to have a background in relationship counseling, psychiatry, psychology or clinical social work. They may even have a medical background, but they will have received specialist training in order to be recognized as a sex therapist qualified to advise individuals or couples on problems within their relationships that are sexually related in some way.

Put simply, a sex therapist treats sex problems with science and an open mind, in the specialized manner that is often required in such cases. Personal opinion and experience are not usually likely to influence the way they work with their patients, and each new case is approached with an open mind, but also with several scientifically proven solutions in mind. Although the treatment is tailored to the individual, it is based on years of experience in the field, and scientific back up. Most sex therapists have a much more detailed knowledge of human physiology as it is affected by sexuality, and all the processes the body goes through before, during and after sexual intercourse. In fact, a really good sex therapist may have more expert knowledge of this particular area of physiology than many medical practitioners.

A sex therapist is not a snake oil salesman or a prostitute or escort under a more job polite description. It's not like in some porn films, where the sex therapist jumps into bed with one, two or several of his or her clients, and everyone's sexual problems are resolved as if by magic with the cameras rolling. In fact, most sex therapy revolves around talk and advice. In a few – very rare – cases, a surrogate partner therapist may be used. We'll take a look at that option later in this chapter, because it's something totally different.

What to expect from a sex therapist

In the initial session, your sex therapist will want you to do most of the talking, so he or she can determine whether the cause of your problem is physical, psychological or a combination of both. Questions will be asked, and you'll need to answer them as fully and as honestly as you can. Depending on the exact details of your personal case, it may take more than one session to complete this important first step.

This detailed assessment will help the sex therapist to formulate a plan of action for you, and decide how often you need to attend therapy sessions. The therapist may suggest that your partner attends some or all of the sessions with you, or you may attend on your own. You will not be expected to do anything against your wishes, and the atmosphere should be relaxed and friendly, to allow you to open up to your therapist and work together to solve your problems.

Part of the therapy will involve doing exercises at home between the sessions, either alone or with your partner. These will be formulated to help you understand your body and your sexuality, and enhance your self confidence and sexual awareness. You should remember – and your therapist should remind you regularly – that sex is supposed to be an enjoyable, pleasurable experience, and the sessions will be geared towards that achievement. Some of the exercises may not seem to have much point, but remember this is a scientific treatment program, and there is a reason for everything you are asked to do. If you don't understand something, ask your therapist to explain, because you need to work together on this if you are to get maximum benefit from the sessions.

You will need to provide a detailed history of your sex life to date. This is not salacious interest on the part of the therapist – it's an excellent way to pinpoint when problems started, and in some cases, why. You'll also need to talk about masturbation, because in a lot of cases of erectile dysfunction – particularly those involving younger men – there is no problem achieving or maintaining an erection, it just happens when they are with a partner. This may mean that performance anxiety is exacerbating your problem, and your therapy will be geared to address this, and any other issues that transpire during the initial assessment. Everything you say to your therapist is and will always remain confidential, so be open and honest, and answer all questions as fully as you can. Talking in this way helps you to understand why you are having problems maintaining erections, as well as teasing out long-buried stuff that you thought you'd forgotten but which may still be impacting on your life, even after many years. It's all very cathartic, and it can help your therapist to formulate the most appropriate and effective program for your needs. Don't be ashamed and hold back on anything – it may be a cliché, but your therapist really has heard it all before. He or she will not be shocked by your revelations, so open up, and let it all out in the presence of someone who is highly trained to help you work through your problems and move on with your life and your sex life.

Although the atmosphere is meant to be relaxed and intimate, inviting confidences, the therapist will not touch you, because what goes on in the office is based around talk, not bodily contact. It's against the professional code of practice to touch clients, and this will be explained to you at the outset. It makes sense when you think about it – it would be only too easy for the client to develop an unhelpful and inappropriate attachment to his therapist, given the nature of the secrets he's shared.

The therapist is also likely to ask about your general life outside the bedroom, because he or she needs to build a picture of you as a complete person in order to offer the best counseling and advice for your particular case. Although sex therapy is a science like medicine, the difference is that it's not also tailored to the individual. There may only be one way to remove an appendix, for example, but there are countless ways to approach the treatment of erectile dysfunction within the scientific framework. And it may be that some of the exercises you are asked to do have nothing to do with sex at all. Nevertheless, they are geared towards helping you to attain a more satisfying sex life. For example, if it emerges that you have a poor body image, you may be advised to join a gym or fit some extra exercise into your routine. Or it might be suggested that you try to build more intimacy with your partner in various ways – maybe by having an evening where you sit and hold hands, talk to each other about your dreams for the future or even touch or caress each other, without attempting to have sex.

One very successful way to re-establish lost intimacy is to lie in bed together naked, touching and cuddling, but not attempting foreplay or sex. Often, the simple act of removing the pressure to have sex can be a big help in solving issues of erectile dysfunction, so the therapist may even advise you not to have sex for a certain period of time, and if this is the case, you should respect the advice, because he or she has been dealing with this sort of stuff for a long time. When the therapist thinks you are ready to have successful and fulfilling sexual intercourse, you will be the first to know!

Other 'homework' may include non-sexual touching exercises and recommended reading. The whole process is geared to help you to get to know yourself and your sexuality on a deeper level, so that you can understand what has happened to you and why, and then work through it and take your relationship to the next, happier and more intimate level.

Many sex therapists say that the saddest thing about their profession is that couples and individuals treat sex therapy as the 'last chance saloon,' when so many of the problems they are presented with can be resolved very quickly and simply, even though they initially appear insurmountable to their clients. Most sexual problems do have a solution, but too often, anger and resentment has built up and it may be too late to save the relationship.

Relationship counseling is a natural part of sex therapy – your therapist needs to determine whether something in the relationship is causing or contributing to your erectile dysfunction. In fact, you can expect to cover all aspects of your life and feelings with your sex therapist. Very often, talking about things that have been bottled up for too long – especially things related to sex and intimacy – is a liberating experience for the client, and a revealing one, and you may often discover ways to improve your situation, simply by talking about them with someone who is giving you their undivided attention. If other methods have failed, maybe sex therapy is worth some of your time and effort in your quest to conquer erectile dysfunction.

Surrogate Partner Therapy (SPT)

Surrogate Partner Therapy was the brainchild of American sex experts Masters & Johnson, and it's been around for around 60 years, although it's only recently become more mainstream, due to media attention and movies like *The Sessions*, which dealt with what has up to know been seen as something that's little short of legalized prostitution, or an affair with a veneer of respectability. However, used in the right way and for the right people, it can help men to overcome erectile dysfunction.

A sex therapist does not offer sex as part of the client's therapy. Indeed professional ethics and common sense decree that no body contact should take between client and therapists during consultations. However, another aspect of sex therapy, which is usually used in conjunction with conventional therapy sessions involve using a surrogate partner who will perform sexual and intimate acts with you as part of the therapy. Not every client is a suitable candidate for this, and not every case is appropriate for surrogate partner therapy.

This is no regular affair, and it's nothing like an encounter with a prostitute – it's a businesslike arrangement in which a highly trained surrogate will work with a client to address and treat their sexual problems in conjunction with conventional sex therapy. At the same time, the surrogate and client form a real relationship and develop the level of intimacy and sharing that is necessary for the surrogate to help the client to achieve his sexual aims and enjoy happy, healthy and fulfilling relationships in the future.

The surrogate may or may not interact sexually with the client, but when that happens, it's not about pleasure in the moment –

it's about dealing with the sexual problem, and helping the client through it by educating him about his body, his sexual and emotional responses and using both structured and unstructured exercises and techniques to overcome the issue of erectile dysfunction.

However, SPT is not all about sex – it's concerned with the whole spectrum of relationships – how you feel about your body, and how you can have a much better, happier and long term relationship with your life partner or partners, with sex, but most of all, and most importantly, with yourself. It may be good to talk, but sometimes talk isn't enough, and people need practical experience in overcoming sex-related issues – if you want to put it a particular way, they need to be shown, rather than advised, how to overcome their sexual difficulties.

Working with a trained partner who is deeply aware of their own sexuality as well as having a specialized knowledge about giving and receiving pleasure can be very rewarding for some people. In the case of erectile dysfunction, this approach may work where others have failed, because there is no pressure to please, even if the pressure is self-imposed. This is a learning experience, and the client will be shown techniques and talked through why some things work and others do not.

SPT is a combination of scientifically developed sexual exercises aimed at rethinking the attitude and developing couples communication so that everything in the bedroom is geared towards mutual pleasure and enjoyment, rather than seeing orgasm as the end objective, and New Age and Eastern thinking on self-awareness and relaxation techniques. You learn to connect mind and body through meditation, relaxation and breathing exercises, combined with practical techniques designed to enhance enjoyment for both partners. This brings about a new self-confidence that is not confined to the bedroom but radiates into all areas of the client's life.

The successful surrogate partner will work to build the same level of intimacy and commitment that exists in regular relationships. This may involve various exercises in touching sexually, sensually and even non-sexually, as well as encouragement and training in social skills, and learning to please a partner and accept intimacy and pleasure unselfconsciously.

Some SPTs claim 85% success in cases of erectile dysfunction, and claim to succeed where conventional therapy and medical intervention have previously failed. Ensure that your potential surrogate has been trained to International Professional Surrogate Association standards and ask lots of questions before committing to an expensive program of treatment. You will also work with a regular sex therapist, and between the three of you, you will decide on boundaries, goals, and the length of your relationship with your surrogate. Yes it's expensive, but you may consider it money well spent if it solves your problems. However, not every man is a suitable candidate for Surrogate Partner Therapy, so it may be better to talk to a conventional sex therapist before pursuing that treatment option.

While sex therapy is not for everyone, it is a viable option for treating erectile dysfunction, because it concentrates on the sexual aspect of your life while also encompassing your relationships and lifestyle. It can be initially embarrassing to discuss such intimate matters, but you could find the experience both empowering and effective. Cost may be a determining factor, since sex therapy, and particularly surrogate partner therapy, can be expensive, and is not usually covered national health services or regular health insurance policies. However, if other options have failed, you may want to try some form of sex therapy to address your erectile dysfunction issues.

Chapter 16

How You Can Still Enjoy Sex with Erectile Dysfunction

As has been mentioned before, one of the acknowledged ways of dealing with erectile dysfunction successfully is to take away the pressure to maintain an erection, by shifting the focus from the orgasm as the main objective of sex. Instead, concentrate on giving and receiving pleasure. There are a number of things you can do to alter your focus. If your partner is understanding, then you can do stuff together, and you can work on your own. Here are some ideas to enjoy sex even if you can't maintain your erection.

Masturbate - alone or together!

You may already have noticed that, even though you can't maintain an erection during sex, you can if you masturbate. That's because there's no pressure to perform – it's just you and your hand, and only you will know if you 'fail.' So maybe you've taken to relieving your frustrations by masturbating, and it's a good call, because it's known to increase the blood flow to the genital area. This is one of the major requirements for a successful and sustainable erection, so it could help you to overcome your erection difficulties.

Why not try mutual masturbation with your partner? This can be a very erotic experience, if you go about it in the right way. Make sure you are warm, comfortable and relaxed, and maybe enjoy some kissing and cuddling first. If you want to use a lubricant – and a good lubricant does stimulate the genitals, and help you to experience a more satisfying orgasm – you could apply it to each other, looking into each other's eyes as you do it, and creating sexual energy before you take responsibility for your own orgasms.

Don't be in any rush to get to the finishing post – take your time, and watch what your partner does with her hands. See where she touches herself for the most arousal, and enjoy the privilege of witnessing her pleasure. Talk to each other, describe in detail how what you are doing feels like, and suggest different places to touch for increased pleasure. Focus on her pleasure, and encourage her to let herself go and enjoy the sensation of masturbating as you watch.

For many men and women, watching their partners come is a great turn on, and makes their own orgasm even more enjoyable, so concentrate on her pleasure, and forget about yourself. You may even find that, by concentrating on your partner, you will be able to maintain your erection and reach orgasm. Each time you manage this, your confidence will increase, and maybe it won't be too long until you can enjoy full penetrative, orgasmic sex again.

In the meantime, mutual masturbation is great fun, and it will become even more so as you become more comfortable with watching each other. If you find you are embarrassed at first, you could try going into different rooms and watching each other on web cam or Skype. It can be very liberating feel slightly wicked, because you're alone, and yet you're not. You could even engage in a little role play if you are both agreeable, and pretend you are strangers having cyber-sex. There's a lot more to mutual masturbation than just making yourself come while you watch your partner have her orgasm.

Oral sex

Oral sex is an excellent way to satisfy your partner without actually having penetrative sex, and you will feel good about satisfying her, so your self-esteem will get a much-needed boost. Try the classic 69 position, and you can also enjoy it, even if you don't actually have an orgasm. Find a position that's comfortable –that could be her on top, you on top, or facing each other sideways. Another way is for you to lie across the bed with your head over the side while she stands over your face, then slides along your body to take your penis in her mouth.

With a 69, whoever is on top is the one in control, so it may be a good idea to let your partner be on top, so you have no other responsibility than to please her with your hands, tongue and mouth. You could well find that with the pressure off, you can indeed get an erection and maintain it, and it should certainly be pleasing for your partner. As has been mentioned more than once in this book, shifting the focus from the end product of an orgasm to the idea of simply giving and receiving pleasure is a great way to relieve the pressure to perform, and thus ease performance anxiety.

The thing about good mutual oral sex is that it teaches you to be more of a participant than a performer, and that's what you need to do to overcome erectile dysfunction. Your penis is part of the whole person, it's not just a pleasure machine you can switch on and off when required.

You may wish to try penetrative sex again after a few successful sessions with oral sex and mutual masturbation. If so, give yourself the best chance of success by making sure the room is comfortable. Taking a warm shower will help to boost the blood circulation and give it the best chance of flowing successfully into your penis and giving you an erection you can maintain. Why not shower with your partner, and make that part of the foreplay?

Again, concentrate on the participation, rather than the performance and the end game.

If you can train yourself to enjoy the moment, eventually you will overcome performance anxiety and learn to love sex again. Until that day arrives – and it will, and probably sooner than you expect – repeat this mantra: Participation is the point – I do not need to perform, and I should not expect myself to perform. Your partner wants a true partner in the bedroom, not just a performing penis. And if she's so superficial that she makes a big deal of it when you can't get an erection, she really isn't worthy of your attention. You should be able to talk to your partner, and allow her to reassure you and work with you to overcome your erectile dysfunction. Remember that, and if your partner is part of the problem, maybe it's time to move on. Now let's take a more detailed look at how you can work with your partner on this, both inside and outside the bedroom.

Bradley Martin

Chapter 17

Working through Erectile Dysfunction with Your Partner's Support

If you are facing erectile dysfunction alone, it's much more difficult to get through it than if you have the love and support of a regular partner who understands what you're going through and with whom you can communicate openly about your hopes, fears and difficulties. They say that a problem shared is a problem halved, and that is certainly true about erectile dysfunction. Men don't like to talk about it, even with other men – make that especially with other men – and they also find it difficult opening up to their partners, but if you can take that first step, you'll have an invaluable ally, and the experience of making this difficult journey together will bring you closer than ever, both sexually and emotionally. Here are some ideas to get your partner onside and win her support.

Reassure her that you still find her attractive

Love and attraction is a big part of sex for most women – they find it difficult to separate the two, and if you've been in a long term relationship and your erectile dysfunction is a recent development, she may think you are falling out of love with her. Even if it's a new relationship, she may think you're not really into her, so before you can communicate effectively, you need to get that out of the way first, to clear up any resentment on her part. The thing is, she may not even realize she's feeling resentful until you actually talk about it, so this is the first step to take.

Compliment her on how she looks, tell her how much you love her, and make sure there's plenty of non-sexual contact to preserve intimacy. This can be difficult, because it's natural to avoid any sort of contact, because your brain is racing ahead of your heart and telling you that if you touch her, kiss her and hold hands, she's sure to want sex, and then you'll disappoint her and yourself all over again. It's all tied in with thinking of your penis as something separate from the rest of you, and not seeing the bigger picture. It's the participation versus performance argument again.

Remember, you're part of a loving couple, and sex is just a part of your relationship. There's a lot more to the two of you than just the bedroom, in fact most of your life together is spent outside the bedroom, so you need to concentrate on that, and the first thing to do is to show your partner how much she is loved and wanted. This will also give her the opportunity to reassure you too, but this particular dialog needs to be opened before you can proceed further with this.

If you or your partner finds it difficult to talk about intimacy, maybe some couples counseling will help to open the dialog. One thing is for sure, this thing is not going to go away if you ignore it, it's something you need to face together and work through, so whether you get talking on your own or with professional help, make sure you do.

Experiment and enjoy each other without penetrative sex

The stuff we talked about in the previous chapter will work a lot better if you can talk about what you both like, and how you feel about mutual masturbation, oral sex, and even using sex toys on each other. In fact, just sitting down and talking about it over a glass of wine or a nice meal in a relaxed way may be a turn on in itself. If you find it easier to talk about your desires openly than your partner does – and many men do – encourage her gently to tell you where she likes to be touched, or even suggest she shows you. Get past that fear of initiating physical contact in case it leads to another failed attempt at sex, and show her that you're willing to experiment on this.

You've assured her it's not about her, but with experimentation, you can tell her and show her that because you love her so much, you want to give her pleasure in other ways. She'll love you for that, and it's a great chance for both of you to be more open about what you would like to happen between you when you are in bed. Often, extended foreplay can be even more satisfying than penetrative sex, because you can synchronize your orgasms, or even enjoy it without an orgasm.

Despite what the media and the porn films would have you believe, mutual orgasms at the same moment through penetrative sex are a rarity, not the norm. Many couples that have no sort of sexual problems at all never experience a mutual orgasm through intercourse alone.

Use this time as an opportunity to try new things, like using sex toys. A couples vibrator such as We-Vibe will give you both extra stimulation, and you can have fun together learning how it works best for both of you. Be positive, and see your erectile dysfunction as an opportunity to connect with your own body and your partner on a new level, rather than the end of your sex life, because that can only happen if you allow it to.

Laugh a lot

Okay, erectile dysfunction is no laughing matter, but neither is it a killer of people or relationships unless you allow that to happen. Try not to take it so seriously, and keep your sense of humor through it all. If your first experiments with sex toys are awkward rather than satisfying, try and laugh about it together. Believe it or not, that will help you create a new level of shared intimacy, if you can laugh about things like that. And if one of you makes unintentional erection-related puns, laugh about that too, rather than trying to cover your embarrassment or taking offence. Hardly anything is so serious that there isn't a lighter side to it, and erectile dysfunction is no exception.

If your partner is unable or unwilling to work with you and support you at this time, you need to face the fact that you may be with the wrong person, and make some difficult decisions, but that is not something we need to discuss here. The thing to hold on to is that erectile dysfunction does not mean the end of your sex life, whatever your age, and neither does it have to dominate your life. There are ways to deal with it, whether you are single or in a relationship, and there is plenty of professional help out there for you if you need it and feel that it is appropriate in your case.

It may be a helpful experience to read blogs written by men who suffer or have suffered from erectile dysfunction. Mostly they are brutally honest but also positive and optimistic. Some men even state that they are pleased they had the problem, because it has helped them to get more in tune with their mind and body, experiment with different sexual techniques and become even closer to their partners as a result. Erectile dysfunction is not the end of your masculinity – it can be a whole new beginning.

How your partner can support you best in dealing with erectile dysfunction

Erectile dysfunction can definitely affect your intimate relationship with your wife or lover. Yes, you have a big part to play in treating the condition because first and foremost, it concerns you. But this battle doesn't have to be a lonely one. Your wife or lover's support can go a long way towards treating erectile dysfunction.

First, your partner can learn as much as she can about erectile dysfunction. Because knowledge is often considered power, knowing more about this condition gives her the power to support you even more, especially when it comes to seeking treatment.

Next, your wife or lover must know how to encourage you and to make you feel you're not fighting this battle alone. She needs to assure you that erectile dysfunction is a medical condition that in most cases, can be easily treated. Another way she can encourage you is by letting you know she understands that it isn't about her attractiveness or desirability. Lastly, she should be able to support you in making healthy lifestyle changes in an effort to treat the condition successfully.

Another way she can support you as you go through this condition is by accompanying you on your medical checkups and treatments. Nothing else speaks of unconditional support than being with you every step of the way.

When a particular treatment method doesn't seem to be working, she can remind you about the many other available options for treating the condition and that you shouldn't give up. This support is invaluable as there'll be times when this condition can be very draining emotionally and you'll need every ounce of morale boosting that you can get.

As for herself, your wife or lover can deal with the situation better by openly expressing how you feel about the situation as well as how much she cares about you. She can also deal with the situation by maintaining a positive outlook, which includes openly discussing how both of you can work together to fulfill each other's needs during this particular season of your relationship.

Bradley Martin

Chapter 18
Acupuncture

Acupuncture is the ancient Chinese art of inserting needles or pricking the skin or tissues with needles for pain alleviation and curing various emotional, mental and physical conditions, including erectile dysfunction. Let's look at some of the great benefits of acupuncture for men in general before diving into its erectile benefits.

First, it helps reduce stress. Men and women have different ways of handling stress but men in general tend to deny being stressed out (machismo effect perhaps?) and acknowledge it only when it's at a dangerously high level. Like Thomas the train, they just keep chugging along. It's probably because most men find it to be a badge of manliness – feeling productive and all. It is such a pig-headed way of thinking about stress that makes many men prone to its ill-effects.

And usually, men go for acupuncture for pain relief. But though acupuncture does help in relieving body pains, it can do so much more than that. It can also help reduce stress levels. The results of a study that was conducted by Dr. Ladan Eshkevari – associate professor at Georgetown University's nursing school – on rats that was published in the Journal of Endocrinology showed that stress hormones of those that were administered electronic acupuncture were lower.

Another acupuncture-related benefit for men is that it can help increase mindfulness. Because men tend to just go chugging along mindlessly at times, they tend to go on autopilot and be disconnected from their bodies. Being still and pausing in the middle of a busy schedule can be beneficial in terms of managing stress. Acupuncture helps men to be still for at least 30 minutes – how can you not be when you have needles poked on your body – and as such, regular acupuncture sessions can help men learn how the art of being still both in mind and in body. It's like forced mediation and relaxation. Such purposeful stillness is a great opportunity to sharpen one's senses and discover different ways of experiencing life, making one more alert and focused in the moment.

Lastly, another benefit for men – should they decide to go for acupuncture – is better sexual performance. Most big pharma companies – as would be expected – try their best to convince men that their only hope for potency salvation is by popping pills in the mouth to make their penises pop up. While their pills can certainly help men deal with erectile dysfunction, they don't necessarily go to the root and often times, just address the symptoms. They can also lead to unwanted side effects for those who aren't predisposed to such pills or are taking other medications that can react negatively with such pills.

Acupuncture can help treat erectile dysfunction in several ways. First, acupuncture can help bring libido back to regular levels and reduce stress, frustration, tension, fear and anger for increased sense of arousal. Second, acupuncture can help improve the health of one's nervous system, increasing arousal and consequently, blood flow to the penis. Third, it has been established that acupuncture can directly improve penile blood flow and help alleviate erectile dysfunction. Lastly, it can help rebalance one's body and release endorphins, which can help a person make do without medications that increase the risk or exacerbate existing erectile dysfunction. As you've learned earlier, some prescription medicines cause erectile dysfunction.

Acupuncture can be a natural and safer alternative for treating erectile dysfunction. A capable acupuncturist will diagnose a patient based on his existing symptoms and medical past, from which he or she will identify the optimal acupuncture points for optimal treatment of the condition. Treatments may range up to 20 sessions (one per week).

What to expect

If it's your first time to experience acupuncture, especially for treating your erectile dysfunction, you may wonder – what should you expect? As with any other competent health professional, the acupuncturist won't go straight away to pricking you with needles on your penis. He or she will first inquire about your lifestyle, health, medical conditions, behaviors and any medications you may be currently taking in order to get a good general assessment of your condition. Among other things, she'll check out your tongue and measure your pulse.

You'll be fully clothed during your acupuncture sessions. The acupuncturist will simply raise your pant leg sleeves, arm sleeves and shirt for leg, arm and stomach needles, respectively. Normally, he or she will play relaxing music so you can rest while the needles remain pricked on your skin for up to 50 minutes. When the session's done and the needles are removed, you'll simply go back to your normal daily routine or plan. In fact, you'll do so with an increased sense of vigor and energy due to the energizing effects of acupuncture. Many people actually fall into deep sleep during the sessions, which is also carried on later at night. The next day, they feel even more energized.

Is there any evidence of acupuncture's efficacy in treating impotence or erectile dysfunction? Yes, several studies have established that already. In particular, let's look at a study conducted in Austria by Paul F. Engelhardt, MD and his colleagues on the effect of acupuncture on physiological erectile dysfunction. The study involved 13 men with an average age of 42 years who suffered from physiological erectile dysfunction. To make sure that these men's impotence weren't just psychological, each men were given "erection" drugs for 3 straight evenings and using what's called a RigiScan testing, all men in the group experienced a full erection and thus, establishing that their erectile dysfunction wasn't psychological. They were split into 2 groups and each group were treated differently.

In the first group, the men were treated with acupuncture for erectile dysfunction while the other group was also given acupuncture treatments but in areas that weren't relevant to treating erectile dysfunction. The objective of using acupuncture on different areas was to determine if a placebo effect was present and strong enough to give patients relief by simply giving them ideas that they're being treated for impotence.

In the first group of 7 men, each underwent 2 acupuncture sessions weekly for 10 weeks on areas that are acupuncture-related for treating erectile dysfunction while the men in the 2nd group (6 men) went through 4 weeks of acupuncture but on areas or acupuncture points that weren't related to treating erectile dysfunction. This group was the placebo group.

The study showed that none of the men in the placebo group experienced erectile dysfunction relief with the placebo treatment and as such, were transferred to the other group or the non-placebo group. At the end of the study, 8 of the 13 men reported that they were cured of their erectile dysfunction and about 2/3 of them reported that the acupuncture therapy yielded good results and didn't demand additional therapy anymore. The remaining 1/3, however, reported that the improvements brought about by the therapy wasn't sufficient that they asked for more therapy and were treated with Viagra.

Another doctor, James Dillard, M.D., said that acupuncture seems to work on an emotional and psychological level in terms of treating erectile dysfunction. He says that as acupuncture sessions make men feel much better about themselves and more relaxed, their erectile dysfunction gets better.

A director at a North Texas urology center, Michael Heltemes opined that acupuncture can possibly help men address their impotence issues and that merely dismissing it as an alternative treatment without adequate evaluation of information may be a disservice for men who are looking for relief from impotence.

Conclusion

Sexual impotence can happen to any man. It doesn't spell any kind of failure on the part of the man, and it can simply be a message from the body to say that something is wrong and needs addressing. Once you address the problems that have arisen, there is no reason why you can't enjoy a full sex life beyond erectile dysfunction.

Listen to what your body is telling you. Don't guess at what the remedies are. Speak to professionals and find out factual information on why your body is not functioning to its optimal levels.

This book has shown you that there is a combination of reasons why this may be happening, but the hope out there is well founded. Even those at an advanced age can still experience erection even if this means employing different methods outlined in this book as a temporary measure while getting the body back into the shape it needs to be in for optimal sexual performance.

The dialog between you and your partner is vital to healing. It is also vital to finding out about each other's trigger points and improves your love life enormously. Men and women don't automatically know all of the answers, but together they are able to find out where their lovemaking techniques need a little more help.

Once you discover the reason, this makes recovery much easier to handle and you and your partner can indeed go on to enjoying a wonderful love life, once all the body's needs are met.